The Politics of the National Health Service
Second Edition

LONGMAN GROUP UK LIMITED,
Longman House, Burnt Mill, Harlow,
Essex CM20 2JE, England

and Associated Companies throughout the world.

Published in the United States of America
by Longman Publishing, New York

© Longman Group UK Limited 1983, 1989

First published 1983
Second edition 1989
Third impression 1992

BRITISH LIBRARY CATALOGUING IN PUBLICATION DATA

Klein, Rudolph, 1930–
  The politics of the National Health Service.—2nd
  ed.
  1. Great Britain. National health service. Political
  aspects
  I. Title
  362.1'0941

ISBN 0-582-03131-1

LIBRARY OF CONGRESS CATALOGING IN PUBLICATION DATA

Klein, Rudolf.
    The politics of the National Health Service/Rudolf Klein.— 2nd
  ed.
      p.   cm.
    Includes index.
    ISBN 0-582-03131-1
    1. National Health Service (Great Britain) 2. Medical policy—
  England. 3. Public health — England. I. Title.
  RA395.G6K64   1989
  362.1'0941— dc20   89-2603
                                                                        CIP

Set in 10/11pt Comp/Set Plantin
Produced by Longman Singapore Publishers (Pte) Ltd.
Printed in Singapore

THE POLITICS OF THE NATIONAL HEALTH SERVICE

Second Edition

Rudolf Klein

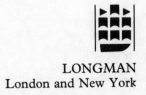

LONGMAN
London and New York

CONTENTS

PREFACE TO FIRST EDITION

Britain's National Health Service is a unique experiment in social engineering. It is the only social service in Britain which is comprehensive in scope in the sense of looking after the entire population. It is, furthermore, the only service that is organised around an ethical imperative: its proclaimed aim is to achieve equity in the distribution and use of health care. Finally, it is remarkable for its sheer size, complexity and heterogeneity: with one million employees, drawn from a variety of professions and representing a wide range of skills, it is the largest employer in the country.

Internationally, too, the NHS is unique. It is the only national health care system, centrally financed and directed, operating in a pluralistic political environment. All other Western societies are characterised by the fact that their pluralistic organisation of health care matches their pluralistic political environment: even Sweden, which comes closest to the British model, delegates responsibility for health care to local government. Similarly, the Communist societies are characterised by the fact that their monopolistic organisation of health care matches the monopolistic political system. Only Britain is different in seeking to have the best of both worlds.

The aim of this book is to explore both the opportunities and the problems which follow from the special characteristics of Britain's NHS. For if the NHS is of interest both to those concerned with specific issues of health care policy-making and to those concerned with the political dynamics of complex modern societies, as I believe it is, the reason is precisely that it can be seen as a laboratory for a whole range of social, institutional and organisational experiments with implications for other areas of policy and other countries.

The NHS illustrates with special sharpness, for example, one of the main policy dilemmas faced by all modern societies: how best to integrate experts into the policy machinery – how to reconcile policy-making seen as the product of political processes and policy-making seen as a search for abstract rationality based on expertise. Again, the NHS's experience underlines the tensions between policies designed to achieve national standards in the pursuit of equity and other policy aims, such as the encouragement of local participation: it can be seen as a case study of conflicting values in the design of social policies. Lastly, the NHS provides an opportunity to study the classic question of political analysis: who gets what? In other words, a health care system can be seen as a political world in its own right, where the balance of power will determine the distribution of resources.

These are some of the main themes running through this book. They are illustrated and elaborated on by analysing the experience of the NHS over the past thirty-five years. For the politics of health care in Britain can best be understood, in my view, as a succession of attempts to solve specific problems and to resolve conflicts of values – with each solution, in turn, creating new problems and conflicts. Some of these problems were built into the original struc-ture of the NHS as it was set up in 1948. Others reflect changes in the economic, political and technological environment. Of course, the political actors involved in this exercise also changed over time. So one of the further aims of the book is to analyse the evolving nature of the health care policy arena.

In all this, it is assumed that the reader does not necessarily come equipped with any knowledge of the NHS. The analytic themes are thus seen as the threads which will help him or her through that complex and confusing labyrinth: Britain's NHS. However, this approach also means that this book is in no sense a history of the NHS. It does not attempt to present a comprehensive picture of events; nor does it attempt to examine all the policy issues or controversies that have arisen over the past thirty-five years. Instead, it is highly selective and concentrates on those issues which seem best to illuminate the analytic themes and to provide the most insight into political processes.

The analysis is also selective in that it deals exclusively with the NHS in England. The organisation of health services in Scotland and Northern Ireland, and to a lesser extent in Wales, differs in some important respects from that in England. So does the style of policy-making: a fact which raises intriguing questions about the relationship between the size of the health care policy arena and the way in which policy is made and implemented. But to have extended the analysis to include the comparative dimension would have added greatly to length, and so reluctantly a Little Englander approach has been adopted.

Throughout, the analysis is informed by interviews with policymakers in central government, in health authorities and in professional and trade union organisations. These interviews were conducted on a 'lobby' basis: that is, on the understanding that the information given was for use but not for attribution. The quotations in the text are therefore not attributed to specific sources. While serving civil servants, and others still involved in policy-making, would probably not thank me for naming them in a list of those who have helped me, I would like to express my gratitude to the following for giving generously of their time: Lord Aberdare; Michael Allison; Barbara Castle; the late Richard Crossman; Douglas Houghton; Sir Alan Marre; Sir Richard Meyjes; Audrey Prime; Kenneth Robinson; Dame Enid Russell-Smith; Dr Derek Stevenson.

Throughout I have tried to quote directly from original sources wherever this was possible, and I am grateful to the Keeper of the Public Record Office for permission to quote Cabinet and other papers. Policy-making is dialogue, and it seems to me important to try to catch the tone of voice, the intellectual style and assumptions used by those involved. In this respect, the analysis of policy-making is rather like the analysis of literature: to paraphrase the documents is to risk losing precisely what gives them their special, unique character.

This book inevitably reflects the intellectual influence and stimulus of those with whom I have discussed the NHS over the years: an influence not fully reflected in the footnotes. Among those who have contributed most to my education are Sir George Godber, Professor T. R. Marmor, Professor J. N. Morris and the late Ron Brown. I am also grateful to Professor Daniel Fox for reading, and commenting on, the manuscript of this book; if I had taken all his advice, it would be a better book. Needless to say, none of those named bears any responsibility for what I have written; I suspect they may disagree strongly with some of my analysis.

Lastly, this book owes much to the help of Dr Renuka Rajkumar, who carried out an analysis of party manifestos and other political sources for me, and Susan Johnson, the Librarian of the Centre for Studies in Social Policy. It certainly would not have been

The politics of the National Health Service

produced at all but for Sylvia Hodges, whose cheerful efficiency in organising me and in typing the manuscript made the completion of this book possible.

University of Bath, December 1982

viii

PREFACE TO SECOND EDITION

I completed the first edition of this book six years, and two General Elections, ago. Since then, the politics of the National Health Service have moved to the centre of the national stage. The political debate has increased in volume and leapt up the scale of partisan acrimony. The consensus which in the past contained party differences seems to have crumbled as the Opposition has made the NHS its chosen battleground. In the circumstances, it was tempting to re-write the final chapters of the book. Instead, I have simply added a new concluding chapter to bring the story up to the beginning of 1989, and this for two reasons. First, I hope it may be illuminating for the reader to see where I was right and wrong in my previous analysis and predictions. Second, despite much turmoil and some change, the 1989 NHS is not so very different from the 1983 NHS in its financial and organisational structure. Its institutional marble has proved remarkably tough, and in many ways it still remains a monument to its original architects.

The new chapter therefore addresses what I see as the central paradox. This is that, while the structure of the NHS has changed remarkably little, the way in which we have come to think about the delivery of health care has changed greatly. In turn, this mirrors a wider revolution in the way we think about the Welfare State and its institutions: the result, as I shall argue, not so much of a decade of Thatcherism as of the underlying social, economic and technological trends which help to explain why Mrs. Thatcher has won three General Elections in a row. It is this transformation in the environment of health care politics – and our collective stock of ideas – which provides the starting point for my second thoughts and the basis for my revised speculations about the future of the NHS: can it continue to evolve within the existing institutional

The politics of the National Health Service

framework in order to adapt to the new environment or will the marble crack as the stresses get too much?

In writing the final chapter, I have drawn on discussion and work done with my colleagues in this country and abroad, in particular Patricia Day, many of whose ideas are incorporated into the text without acknowledgment. And, as before, I would like to acknowledge the help of the many (necessarily anonymous) civil servants and NHS managers who have helped me to understand the dynamics of the policy process. Finally, my thanks to Mrs. Janet Bryant for organising me and my typing.

The first edition of this book came out in the 'Politics Today' series, edited by Bernard Crick and Patrick Seyd. I am most grateful to the former in particular for his encouragement and for being a more tolerant editor than I was when our roles were reversed.

University of Bath, February 1989

Chapter one
THE POLITICS OF CREATION

If many simultaneously and variously directed forces act on a given body, the direction of its motion cannot coincide with any of those forces, but will always be a mean – what in mechanics is represented by the diagonal of a parallelogram of forces. If in the descriptions given by historians . . . we find their wars and battles carried out in accordance with previously formed plans, the only conclusion to be drawn is that those descriptions are false.

Leo Tolstoy, *War and Peace*

Britain's National Health Service (NHS) came into existence on 5 July 1948. It was the first health system in any Western society to offer free medical care to the entire population. It was, furthermore, the first comprehensive system to be based not on the insurance principle, with entitlement following contributions, but on the national provision of services available to everyone. It thus offered free and universal entitlement to State-provided medical care. At the time of its creation it was a unique example of the collectivist provision of health care in a market society. It was destined to remain so for almost two decades after its birth when Sweden, a country usually considered as a pioneer in the provision of welfare, caught up. Indeed, it could be held up as 'the greatest Socialist achievement of the Labour Government', to quote Michael Foot, the biographer of Aneurin Bevan who, as Minister of Health in that Government, was the architect of the NHS.[1]

The transformation of an inadequate, partial and muddled patchwork of health care provision into a neat administrative structure was dramatic, even though the legislative transformation was built on the evolutionary developments of the previous decades. At a legislative stroke, 1,000 hospitals owned and run by a large variety of voluntary bodies and 540 hospitals operated by local authorities were nationalised. At the same time, the benefits of free general practitioner care, hitherto limited to the 21 million people covered by the insurance scheme originally set up by Lloyd George in 1911, were extended to the entire population. From then on, everyone was entitled, as of right, to free care – whether provided by a general practitioner or by a hospital doctor – financed by the State. At the summit of the administrative structure there was the Minister of Health. Under the terms of the 1946 Act setting up the NHS, the Minister was charged with the duty 'to promote the establishment in England and Wales of a comprehensive health service designed to secure improvement in the physical and mental health of the people of England and Wales and the prevention, diagnosis and treatment of illness, and for that purpose to provide or secure the effective provision of services'. The services so provided, the Act further laid down, 'shall be free of charge'.

How did this transformation come about? It is not the aim of this chapter to provide a history of the creation of the NHS: other sources are available, giving a detailed blow by blow account of what happened in the years leading up to 1948.[2] The intention, rather, is to analyse the political dynamics of the creation: to identify the main groups of actors in the arena of health care politics and to delineate the world of ideas in which the plans for a national health service evolved. In doing so, it is necessary to explore the complex interplay between the ineluctable pressure on politicians and administrators to do something about the practical problems forced on to their agenda by the clamouring inadequacies of health care in Britain, as it had evolved over the previous century up to 1939, and their resolution of the policy puzzles involved in accommodating competing values and insistent pressure groups. It was the historical legacy which made it inevitable that *a* national health service would emerge by the end of the Second World War. It was the ideological and practical resolution of the policy puzzles which determined the precise shape taken by the NHS as it actually emerged in 1948.

THE EMERGING CONSENSUS

First, let us examine the nature of the consensus that had emerged by 1939: the movement of ideas which made it seem inevitable that some kind of national health service would eventually emerge – dictated, as it were, by the logic of circumstances, rather than by the ideology of politicians or the demands of pressure groups. Basically, this consensus embodied agreement on two linked assumptions. These were that the provision for health care in Britain, as it had grown up over the decades, was both inadequate and irrational. Health care, it was agreed, was inadequate in terms both of coverage and of quality. Lloyd George's 1911 legislation had provided insurance coverage only for general practitioner services. In turn this coverage was limited to manual workers, excluding even their families. Hospital care was provided by municipal and voluntary institutions on the basis of charging those who could afford to pay and giving free care to those who could not. Even though the bewildering mixture of State insurance, private insurance and the availability of free care in the last resort meant that everyone had access to some form of medical treatment, the quality varied widely. The general practitioner, operating usually on the small shopkeeper principle of running his own practice single-handed and relying mainly on the income from the capitation fees of his insured patients, was isolated from the mainstream of medicine. 'It is disturbing to find large numbers of general practitioners being taught at great trouble and expense to use modern diagnostic equipment, to know the available resources of medicine and to exercise judgement as between patient and specialist', the 1937 Political and Economic Planning (PEP) survey of health care in Britain commented,[3] 'only to be launched out into a system which too often will not permit them to do their job properly'. In the case of the hospital sector, the quality of specialist care varied greatly; indeed there was no officially agreed definition of who should be considered a specialist – the title of consultant being attached to specific posts, mostly in the prestigious teaching hospitals, rather than being a generally accepted description of doctors with special skills recognised according to explicit criteria. In many of the smaller voluntary hospitals, especially, it was general practitioners who carried out both medical and surgical procedures, with no check on their qualifications or competence for the job.

The system, it was further agreed, was irrational. Specialists gravitated to those parts of the country where the population was prosperous enough to pay for private care, since hospital consultancies were honorary and they were thus dependent on income from private practice. By definition, the most prosperous parts of the country were not necessarily those which generated most need for medical care. Voluntary and municipal hospitals competed with, and against, each other. The distribution of beds across the country was determined by historical hazard, not the logic of the distribution of illness: Birmingham, for example, had 5.7 beds per 1,000 population, while Liverpool had 8.6. Hospitals shuffled off responsibility for patients to each other: the voluntary hospitals regularly dumping chronic cases onto the municipal sector. Municipal hospitals could, and indeed did, refuse admission to patients coming from outside their local authority area. A further article of faith in the emerging consensus was, therefore, the need to co-ordinate the various systems – voluntary and municipal – that had emerged, and to introduce some rationality into the distribution of resources.

The consensus had another ingredient. There was widespread acceptance of the fact that the voluntary hospital system was no longer viable financially. By the mid 1930s traditional forms of fundraising from the public – the appeal to altruistic charitable instincts – were not yielding anything like enough to support their activities: only 31 per cent of the income of London Teaching Hospitals and 20 per cent of the income of the provincial teaching hospitals came from this source. More important was income from charges to patients, financed – on a 50 : 50 basis – either out of their own income or out of contributory insurance schemes. The bankruptcy of the voluntary sector was staved off by the Second World War, when these hospitals drew large-scale benefits from the Government's scheme of paying for stand-by beds for war casualties. But it was clear that, in the long term, their dependence on public finance was both irremediable and likely to increase.[4] Equally, it had long since become clear that the original purpose of the most prestigious of the voluntary hospitals – to provide free care for the poor – could not be fully carried out, since financial pressures were forcing them to rely on attracting precisely those patients who could afford to pay. The price of survival was, to an extent, the repudiation of the inspiration which had led to their creation in the first place.

Not surprisingly therefore, the years between the two world wars – between 1918 and 1939 – were marked by the publication of a series of reports from a variety of sources, all sharing the same general perspective. In 1920 the Minister of Health's Consultative Council on Medical and Allied Services (the Dawson report) enunciated the principle that 'the best means of maintaining health and curing disease should be made available to all citizens' – a principle to be later echoed by Aneurin Bevan when he introduced the 1946 legislation – and elaborating this principle in a detailed scheme of organising health care; a hierarchy of institutions starting from the Primary Health Centre and culminating in the Teaching Hospital.[5] In 1926 the Royal Commission on National Health Insurance came to the conclusion, although it balked at spelling it out in its immediate recommendations, that 'the ultimate solution will lie, we think, in the direction of divorcing the medical service entirely from the insurance system and recognising it along with all other public health activities as a service to be supported from the general public funds'.[6] In 1930 the British Medical Association (BMA) came out in favour of extending the insurance principle to the dependents of the working population and supported a co-ordinated reorganisation of the hospital system, while in 1933 the Socialist Medical Association added its radical treble to the conservative bass drum of the BMA and published its plan for a comprehensive, free and salaried medical service, to be managed by local government but with a regional planning tier.[7]

There are a number of strands within this consensus which need disentangling. In the first place, the consensus speaks with the accents of what might be called rationalist paternalists, both medical and administrative. This is the voice not so much of those outraged by social injustice as of those intolerant of muddle, inefficiency and incompetence: a tradition going back to the days of Edwin Chadwick, via the Webbs. It is further, the voice of practical men of affairs, trying to find solutions to immediate problems. In the second place, the consensus reflects a view of health care which was rooted in British experience, though not unique to it: an intellectual bias which helps to explain why the institutional solution devised in the post-war era was unique to Britain.

The second point requires elaboration. When, confronted by the muddle of health care, men started thinking about possible solutions, they had before them two models – either of which could have been developed into a fully-fledged national system. The first model was that of Lloyd George's insurance scheme for general practice: an import from Bismarck's Germany. In theory, there was no reason why such a model could not have been elaborated into a comprehensive national insurance scheme: the road followed by nearly all other Western societies in the post-war period, and advocated by the BMA not only in the 1930s but also subsequently (see Ch. 3). The other model, however, was that of the public health services, developed and based on local authority provision in Britain in the nineteenth century: a model based on seeing health as a public good rather than as an individual right. While the first model emphasised the right of individuals to medical care – a right to be based, admittedly, on purchasing the appropriate insurance entitlements – the second model emphasised the obligation of public authorities to make provision for the health of the community at large. While the first model was consistent with individualistic medical values – given that the whole professional ethos was to see medical care in terms of a transaction between the individual patient and the individual doctor – the second model was consistent with a collectivist approach to the provision of health care. Indeed throughout it is important to keep in mind the distinction between medical care in the strict sense (that is, care and intervention provided by doctors with the aim of curing illness) and health care in the larger sense (that is, all those forms of care and intervention which influence the health of members of the community).

Thus the whole logic of the Dawson report was based on the proposition that 'preventive and curative medicine cannot be separated on any sound principle. They must likewise be both brought within the sphere of the general practitioner, whose duties should embrace the work of both communal as well as individual medicine'. Nor was this just a matter of intellectual tradition. Local government was already in the business of providing health care, ranging from curative medicine in its hospitals to chronic care for the elderly and mentally ill in its institutions, from the provision of maternity clinics to looking after the health of schoolchildren. Organisational bias thus reinforced intellectual bias in the sense that the services provided by local government would have to be incorporated into any national scheme that might emerge. To have adopted an insurance-based scheme would therefore have meant actively repudiating the service-based legacy of the past.

Given this convergence of views on the necessity of devising some form of national health service, as distinct from some form of national health insurance, it is tempting to interpret the eventual emergence of the 1948 NHS in a deterministic fashion: to see it as the child not of Labour ideology, not as a Socialist triumph, but as the inevitable outcome of attempts to deal with a specific situation in the light of an intellectual consensus, both about what was desirable and about what was possible. Equally, given this convergence, it would seem redundant to search for explanations in Britain's wartime experience, whether administrative or emotional. The acceptance of the need for a national health service long predates, as we have seen, the wartime administrative experience of running the emergency medical service: an experience which, at best, can have generated confidence that it was actually possible to run a complex web of hospitals and services. Similarly, this acceptance long predates the wartime commitment to a collectivist solution of welfare problems: a commitment epitomised in the 1942 Beveridge report which assumed, without elaborating in detail, the creation of a 'comprehensive national health service'.

Accepting a general notion is, of course, one thing. Devising and implementing a specific plan is, however, a very different matter. The consensus may have provided a foundation. It did not provide a blueprint: when it came to detail, the various proposals put forward during the inter-war period had all come up with somewhat different schemes. To examine the evolution of plans from the outbreak of war in 1939 to the enactment of the 1946 legislation for setting up the National Health Service is to identify a whole series of clashes not only between interest groups but also between competing values. If everyone was agreed about the end of policy in a general sort of way, there was little by way of consensus about means – and much awareness of the fact that the means chosen might, in turn, affect the end. It was a conflict of a peculiar sort: conflict contained, and limited, by an overarching consensus – a constraint which forced compromise and caution on all the protagonists. Indeed, as we shall find, the theme of conflict within consensus is one which runs through the entire history of the NHS.

THE CURTAIN GOES UP

An appropriate starting point for tracing the evolution of policy is a memorandum written only a few days after the outbreak of the Second World War, on 21 September 1939 by the Ministry of Health's Chief Medical Officer, Sir Arthur MacNalty. This formed part of a series of papers[8] prepared for discussion by a small group of civil servants who, already in 1938, had started considering the future development of health services. At the first meeting, the Permanent Secretary – Sir John Maude – had outlined two possible lines of approach: 'either the gradual extension of National Health Insurance to further classes of the community and by new statutory benefits, or the gradual development of local authority services.' But in his memorandum, MacNalty addressed himself to a third option: 'the suggestion that the hospitals of England and Wales should be administered as a National Hospital Service by the Ministry.'

Since it was precisely this suggestion which prevailed – in so far as the 1948 NHS was, essentially, a national hospital service – it is worth examining MacNalty's arguments in some detail. First, he pointed out that a National Hospital System 'is already practically established for purposes of a national emergency'. Second, he argued that 'it will be difficult and in many cases be impossible for voluntary hospitals to carry on owing to the high costs of modern hospital treatment and the falling off of voluntary subscriptions after the war'. But then, turning to the case against such a solution, MacNalty outlined the possible objections. First, 'the nationalisation of the hospitals would dry up the flow of voluntary subscriptions which largely contribute to relieving the ratepayer and the taxpayer of the cost of hospital provision'. Second, 'the majority of the medical profession would be bitterly opposed to it. This would cause much dissension, controversy and ill-feeling at a time when it is vitally important that national unity should be preserved'. Third, the proposal implied 'a radical change in the policy of the Ministry. Hitherto, we have always worked on the assumption that the Ministry of Health was an advisory, supervisory and subsidising department, but had no direct executive functions'. Lastly, 'from the point of view of local authorities executive control of all hospitals by the State might excite opposition and present difficulties'.

In conclusion, however, MacNalty came out on the side of nationalisation, if only tentatively. He wrote:

It is a revolutionary change, but it is one that must inevitably come, because the voluntary system with all its excellent attributes is unsuited to the modern needs of the whole population. . . . As I have mentioned, the proposal may meet with much opposition from the medical profession. But I am certain they would, for the most part, welcome national control in preference to being controlled by local authorities. We have a very good method of approach to them in showing that even before the war the voluntary system was breaking down, that it has failed in wartime to cope with modern conditions and has necessitated general hospital control by the State. I suggest then the time is ripe that we should approach the medical profession in this way, not as seeking to impose a national system upon them, but taking them into council, saying, for example, these are our difficulties. Will you help us find a way out of them? On these lines it might be possible to get a National Hospital Service established by negotiation with the general agreement and support of the medical profession.

There was, of course, yet a further option, discussed in a memorandum written the subsequent day by Sir Arthur Rucker – a senior civil servant, later to be the Ministry's Deputy Secretary. As between the Permanent Secretary's option of municipalisation and the Chief Medical Officer's option of nationalisation, there was the possibility of establishing a mixed economy system. This could be done by establishing 'joint hospital boards', which would be responsible for planning both municipal and voluntary hospital services.

Financial support to the voluntary hospitals would be contingent on them co-operating. The advantage of such an approach, Rucker argued, was that it offered the 'most practical solution' since it would build on existing developments. Further, it would avoid the administrative problems of nationalisation: 'We simply have not the medical or administrative staff that could cope with so enormous a task and it is difficult to see how such a staff could be recruited from outside the Ministry at the present moment.'

So here, in 1939 already, we have set out most of the main assumptions, issues and factors that shaped the discussions over the next six years, in so far as they affected hospital as distinct from general practitioner services, at any rate. The exchange of notes is revealing in a number of respects. It shows civil servants taking the initiative in generating policy options unprompted, as far as can be judged from the records, by the politicians. It also indicates their operating assumptions: the emphasis is on seeking 'practical' solutions which will be acceptable, on bringing about change through agreement. It reveals the bias of the Ministry of Health: a department with a tradition of regulatory rather than executive functions, reluctant to take on direct administrative responsibilities for a complex service. It shows the natural inclination of civil servants to build on existing developments and organisations, rather than to invent new institutions. However, it also shows a civil service engaged in a wide-ranging search operation, as it examines a wide range of possible policies: if the style is evolutionary, radical solutions are not excluded.

But these notes not only define the rules of the game, as interpreted by the Ministry of Health hierarchy. They also define the arena of health care politics: those considered to be legitimate actors, with a claim to participate in the negotiations. The cast-list is as significant for those left out as it is for those included. Among the excluded are the Approved Societies which administered the existing national insurance system: an exclusion all the more notable given the dominant role of these societies in the formation of the system in the period between 1911 and 1913.[9] So, too, are the majority of those actually working in health services: from nurses to floor sweepers. But included are the voluntary hospitals, local authorities and, above all, the medical profession. The key to successful change is seen to be, as is clear from MacNalty's memorandum, the support and co-operation of the medical profession. Even allowing for the fact that as Chief Medical Officer, and thus the middleman between the Ministry and the profession, MacNalty was bound to put particular stress on the role of doctors, this is a recurring theme. It is further reflected in the records of the Ministry over the next few years: records which document a seemingly endless series of meetings between Ministry officials and representatives of the medical profession, as well as with the voluntary hospital and other interests.

One set of characters remains to be introduced: the politicians – the political masters of the Ministry of Health. This late introduction of what might be expected to be the central actors may seem perverse in a book devoted to the politics of health. In fact, however, it is entirely appropriate. For most of the time in the period covered, politicians play the role of Fortinbras: when he comes on stage in the last scene, the trumpets may sound – but all the protagonists of the action are dead. Only occasionally, and exceptionally, do the politicians play a central role in the drama. The point is well illustrated by the evolution of policy between 1939 and 1946: a story which breaks into two sharply distinguished sections – the politics of compromise under the Coalition Government, during which politicians are fringe figures, and the politics of innovation under the Labour Government, when politicians take the centre of the stage.

COALITION COMPROMISES

The best starting point for considering the evolution of policy under the wartime Coalition Government is to examine the end-product of the years of negotiation: the 1944 White Paper setting out the plans for a National Health Service,[10] written by Sir John Hawton, subsequently the Ministry of Health's Permanent Secretary. This was based upon two principles, which were to remain the foundation of the National Health Service as it finally emerged in 1946. First, that the new service should be comprehensive: that 'every man and woman and child can rely on getting all the advice and treatment and care which they need . . . . and that what they get shall be the best medical and other facilities available'. Second, that the service should be free: that 'their getting these shall not depend on whether they can pay for them, or on any other factor irrelevant to the real need – the real need being to bring the country's full resources to bear upon reducing ill-health and promoting good health in all its citizens'.

Although the proclaimed ends of the 1944 White Paper were the same as those of the 1946 Act, yet the institutional means were different. As the White Paper argued, there were two alternative strategies for achieving change: 'One, with all the attraction of simplicity, would be to disregard the past and the present entirely and to invent *ad hoc* a completely new reorganisation for all health requirements. The other is to use and absorb the experience of the past and the present, building it into the wider service.' It was the second approach which shaped the White Paper, not surprisingly perhaps given the fact that the Minister of Health, Henry Willink, was a Conservative and given also the intellectual bias of the civil servants.

More important still the White Paper was an attempt to reconcile the views of the principle coalition partners: the Conservative and Labour parties. When the Prime Minister, Winston Churchill, had last-minute qualms about publishing the White Paper, he got a sharp reminder about the political realities from Lord Woolton, the Minister for Reconstruction.[11] The latter pointed out:

This is a compromise scheme, but it is a compromise which is very much more favourable to the Conservatives than to Labour Ministers and when it is published, I should expect more criticism from the Left than from Conservative circles.... If discussion of the whole scheme is to be re-opened. . . . I fear that the Labour Ministers may withdraw their support of the scheme and stand out for something more drastic which would be far more repugnant to Conservative feeling.

The White Paper was also an attempt to minimise opposition from the various interest groups in the arena of health care politics. Indeed any solution would be politically acceptable to the extent that it avoided a clash with those interests, particularly since each of these tended in turn to have their links with the political parties: a link which was, for example, strong in the case of the Conservative Party and the voluntary hospital movement. To a large extent the records of the negotiations that took place in the years before the publication of the White Paper, as reflected in the files of the Ministry of Health, show the civil servants and the representatives of the three major interest groups (in particular, the medical profession), engaged in searching out the limits of the acceptable: trying to identify the sticking points in each other's position and to devise ways of reconciling the different points of view.

Lastly, though, the White Paper was an attempt to solve certain basic dilemmas of policy. It was a compromise document because it sought to reconcile various aims of policy, all desirable in themselves, which pointed in different directions. It thus incorporated judgements both about the relative weights to be given to considerations of feasibility (maximising political agreement within the Government, minimising opposition from interest groups) and different policy values.[12] So perhaps the most illuminating way of analysing the White Paper proposals is to look at them in the context of the specific dilemmas – the kind of choices between competing tactical considerations and policy aims – faced by those involved in producing the document: dilemmas which provide themes running through the entire history of the NHS, and which still provide an agenda for political debate in the 1980s.

First was the dilemma of how to reconcile government acceptance of the principle of national responsibility for the health care system and the desire to avoid a centralised service actually operated by the Ministry of Health. Not only did the Ministry, as already noted, lack both the experience and the inclination to engage in such an exercise. But, implicit in the debate, was also the further question of the appropriate balance between central and local government, between bureaucratic control from the centre and freedom at the periphery to respond to local demands. Here the White Paper's solution was to assign responsibility for planning the service to the Minister, but executive responsibility to local government which could maintain its function of running hospitals and providing personal health services.

This solution, however, only created a second dilemma. Devolution of responsibility to the periphery assumes the existence of administrative units which are appropriate, in terms of their boundaries and size, to deliver a particular kind of service. In the case of health services, it was generally agreed, the existing structure of local government was inappropriate. In particular, the administrative division between town and country created problems, since the major hospital resources tended to be concentrated in the former. So here the solution was to propose the creation of 30–35 joint authorities, as foreshadowed in Rucker's 1939 memorandum, combining counties and country boroughs, though the option of other permutations of combined local authorities was left open. It would be the responsibility of the new joint authorities to assess the needs of their areas and to plan 'how those needs should best be met'. The plans would, in turn, have to be submitted to and approved by the Ministry of Health (a scheme of things which foreshadows the 1974 reorganisation of the NHS, as we shall see). The new joint authorities would be directly responsible for running hospital and consultant services; responsibility for local clinics and other personal health services would remain with the existing local authorities. The overall objective would be to 'unify and co-ordinate the service' by means of a 'rational and effective plan'.

Third, however, was the dilemma of how it would be possible to devise a 'rational and effective plan' if the voluntary hospitals were left outside the system. Was there a middle way between a national and a pluralistic system? Here the solution was to make government financial help to the voluntary sector dependent on their joining in the planning exercise, a proposal which can also be traced back to Rucker's 1939 memorandum. The joint authorities would be in a contractual relationship with the voluntary section 'for the performance of agreed services set out in the plan' – a scheme which appears to be a direct descendant of Rucker's ideas put forward in 1939. The local plans would cover the totality of resources within any given area, irrespective of their actual ownership. The Minister's control over the system would, in addition, be strengthened by the creation of a hospital inspectorate.

Fourth was the dilemma of how to reconcile public accountability and professional participation in decision-making. The basic principle enshrined in the White Paper was that 'effective decisions on policy must lie entirely with elected representatives answerable to the people for the decisions that they take' – the local government councillors. But the medical profession demanded representation for its views in the formulation of policy, and there was general agreement that the voice of expertise should be heard. The White Paper sought to resolve this dilemma by establishing a Central Health Services Council to advise on national policy and equivalent local bodies to advise on local policy: in short, it established a hierarchy of professional expertise parallel to the institutional hierarchy of public accountability through elected representatives.

Fifth was the dilemma of how to integrate hospital and general practitioner services.[13] If the aim of policy was to secure more efficiency and rationality, it was impossible to exclude general practitioners from the planning process. In particular, as the White Paper stressed, there had to be an effective means of 'ensuring a proper distribution of doctors'. The logic of such an approach pointed in the direction of making general practitioners employees of local authorities. The logic of political feasibility, of minimising opposition, pointed in the opposite direction, however, since the medical profession – through the BMA – was fiercely opposed to such a solution. So here the White Paper proposed to abolish the local Insurance Committees, which had administered general practice since 1913 and were composed of medical representatives as well as lay members. The responsibilities of the Committees would be transferred to a Central Medical Board, which would be responsible for planning the distribution of doctors: thus it would have the power to refuse consent to a general practitioner to practice in areas considered to have a sufficiency of doctors.

Sixth, there still remained the dilemma of how to reconcile the inherited system of general practice based on individualistic, small-shopkeeper principles, with the aim of promoting 'developments in the modern technique of medical practice'. The system of capitation payments encouraged competition between general practitioners: the more patients they had, the bigger their income. Further, the less they spent on equipping their surgeries, the greater was their take-home pay. Yet there was widespread agreement that the quality of general practice could only be improved by groups of general practitioners practising in well-equipped premises, a view in whose support the White Paper could even invoke the 1942 Interim Report of the BMA's Medical Planning Commission. So how was the demand for a new pattern of service to be reconciled with an inherited system of payment which seemed to be in contradiction with the aims of policy? Here the White Paper again proposed a compromise: a compromise which reflected the extreme hostility of the BMA to any proposal which appeared to turn general practitioners into public servants. General practitioners would be encouraged to group themselves in Health Centres to be provided by the new joint local authorities, though they would be employed by the Central Medical Board: the method of payment was left for future decisions, though the White Paper argued that 'there is a strong case for basing future practice in a Health Centre on a salaried remuneration or some similar alternative which does not involve mutual competition'. But other general practitioners would continue in independent practice. The principles of free choice of doctors by patients and complete medical autonomy were to remain sacrosanct.

Like all compromise proposals designed to reconcile multiple and conflicting objectives, the White Paper left most of the actors involved feeling dissatisfied. For all of them, the final compromise left them to tot up a complex balance sheet of gains and losses: the White Paper indeed was a triumph mainly for those, in particular the civil servants, whose prime objective lay precisely in achieving some kind of compromise formula which, even if it did not satisfy any of the actors fully, at least minimised the chances of continued conflict. The medical profession had reconciled itself to accepting a comprehensive health service, abandoning its earlier insistence on limiting coverage to 95 per cent of the population and thus institutionalising the scope for private practice. Again, the medical profession had lost its battle to make the Central Health Services Council representative of the medical profession – an elected rather than a nominated body – which would have an actively directing role in the operations of the health service. But it had successfully fought off the threat of direct local authority control over general practice, and it managed to compel the Coalition Government to produce a fudged formula on the vexed question of payments.

The local government lobby had averted the danger of nationalisation, but was left dissatisfied by the prospect of the new joint authorities actually taking over control of their hospitals: Herbert Morrison, the Home Secretary and the voice of local government in the administration, warned the War Cabinet's Reconstruction Committee that the 'proposed arrangements would undoubtedly be criticised by local authorities'. The voluntary hospitals, too, were unhappy: although they would nominally maintain their independence, they believed that they would suffer a 'mortal blow through the cessation of income from patients', as the Minister of Health told the Reconstruction Committee.[14]

The White Paper also embodied compromises by the political partners in the Coalition Government. Labour Ministers continued to grumble to the last during the sessions of the Reconstruction Committee involved in the final drafting of the White Paper about conceding the right to private practice for general practitioners in the public service. 'There would be a danger that some doctors would devote their energies to maintaining their private practice at the expense of their public patients', Clement Attlee, the leader of the Labour Party, pointed out. The Minister of Labour, Ernest Bevin, argued that the 'White Paper did not sufficiently emphasise the need for a vigorous development of Health Centres, served by a salaried medical staff'. Again, Labour Ministers had been forced to accept a postponement of any decision about the controversial issue of the buying and selling of practices, and whether or not this right should be expropriated.

Similarly, Conservative Ministers had been pushed into accepting policies which, once their Labour partners had left the Coalition Government, they were quick to change. In June 1945, the Cabinet accepted a revised policy programme devised by Henry Willink with the aim of modifying 'certain features in the original plan which had been unpopular with local authorities, voluntary hospitals and the medical profession'.[15] First, there was a major concession to the medical profession. The proposal for a Central Medical Board was dropped, for this had always been regarded with extreme suspicion by the medical profession, who saw it as an attempt by the central bureaucracy to gain control. The local Insurance Committees, though re-titled, were reinstated. Finally, the power to prevent general practitioners from moving into well-provided areas was dropped; instead, distribution was to be improved by offering 'positive inducement by more attractive terms in less attractive areas'. Health Centres were to be experimental only; doctors working in them were to be paid on the same basis as independent general practitioners – that is, by capitation fees. Local authorities were also placated: the new joint authorities were to be limited to the planning function, with control over hospitals left with the existing units of local government.

Finally, the most prestigious of the voluntary hospitals were given a concession they had long sought: in order to give 'the principal medical teaching centres . . . a suitable place in the machinery for co-ordinating the specialised services', it was proposed to set up 'expert regional bodies' to advise on the planning of services. This was, of course, not only a gesture towards the Teaching Hospitals. It was also a response to the arguments of what might be called the 'medical technocracy': those whose concern had long been to achieve a more rational structure of services in terms of the quality of medical care – a concern which can be found in many of the documents published between the wars and which was reinforced during the war by a series of inquiries, sponsored by the Nuffield Provincial Hospitals Trust, into the state and distribution of health resources.[16] If the logic of the joint authorities was the need to make some sort of sense of the existing local government structure, the logic of the regional bodies was the need to plan the more specialised medical services – particularly consultant services – on a larger scale than the administrative units produced by the amalgamation of existing local authorities. The functional geography of local government, it was clear, did not necessarily coincide with the functional geography of the health service: a dilemma which, once again, provides a further theme for the history of the NHS over the next decades.

Within two months of getting the Conservative Cabinet's agreement to his revised proposals, Willink had been replaced by Aneurin Bevan as Minister of Health: a Labour Government, with a triumphant majority, had swept into office. The fragile consensus which had constrained Labour Ministers in the Coalition Government appeared to be shattered. The way was open for the politics of ideology to take over from the politics of compromise.

PRIVATE NEGOTIATION INTO PUBLIC CONTROVERSY

In retrospect, the most remarkable aspect of the controversies that attended the enactment of the National Health Services Bill in 1946 and the setting up of the National Health Service in 1948 is the disparity between the anger generated and the actual changes introduced by Aneurin Bevan. In a sense, the virulent hostility of Bevan's critics – both on the Conservative benches in Parliament and among the medical profession – flattered his achievement and exaggerated the extent to which he broke with the sedimentary consensus that had been built up over the preceding years. From today's perspective, the 1946 legislation was as remarkable for the degree of continuity it represented as for its departures from the agreed compromises of the Coalition Government. In turn, the departures from the agreed compromises reflected as much a defeat for some of Bevan's own colleagues in the Labour Cabinet as an assertion of Socialist ideology at the expense of Conservative ideology.

It is tempting to argue, indeed, that it was in the political interests of everyone concerned to overstate the extent of disagreement. For Bevan, Opposition was a testimonial to his own radicalism; and for the opposition, and the medical profession, it was an opportunity to wash their hands in public over some of the compromises they had accepted during the years of private negotiation. It was Bevan's style of self-presentation – the aggressive insistence that it was the Labour Government's duty to present its proposals to Parliament, rather than hammering them out in private conclave with the representatives of the interest groups – which not only brought the latter's latent suspicions and resentments to the surface, but also gave them the pretext for adopting a stance of public hostility. Compromises which might just about be acceptable as part of an agreed package no longer were so once the package itself had been unwrapped by the Minister without consultation. Indeed this interpretation is strengthened by the otherwise very curious contrast between the relatively easy passage given to Bevan's most radical proposal, that for the hospital service, and the long-drawn-out battle over general practice, where Bevan in fact hardly departed from the previously agreed compromise. It is therefore helpful to consider these two facets of the 1946 legislation separately.

Bevan's plan represented one dramatic break with the immediate past – to the extent that it represented a return to MacNalty's 1939 proposal. His entire scheme was based on 'the complete takeover

– into one national service – of both voluntary and municipal hospitals', as his October 1945 memorandum to the Cabinet put it.[17] In turn this would mean, Bevan's memorandum continued, 'the concentration in the Ministry of Health of responsibility for a single hospital service, coupled with the delegation of day to day administration to new regional and local bodies appointed by the Minister (after consultation with the appropriate local organisations) and responsible to him.' Equally, it would imply 'the centralising of the whole finance of the country's hospital system, taking it right out of local rating and local government'.

In other words, the dilemma of combining national responsibility with responsiveness to local need was to be resolved in a way totally different to that envisaged in the 1944 White Paper: there was to be no split of responsibilities between central and local government, but an attempt to solve the problem of achieving an appropriate balance between the centre and periphery by a process of delegation. It was a solution which was immediately challenged within the Labour Cabinet. The arguments involved deserve close attention, since once again they have continued throughout the history of the NHS and the issue of the appropriate balance between centre and periphery continues to be a major political issue in the 1980s.

The main opposition to Bevan came from Herbert Morrison, Lord President of the Council and, as in the days of the Coalition Government, the voice of local government. In his counter-memorandum to Bevan's,[18] Morrison argued that the Minister of Health is

on the horns of a dilemma. If the Regional Boards and District Committees are to be subject to the Minister's directions on all questions of policy, they will be mere creatures of the Ministry of Health, with little vitality of their own . . . . Yet it is difficult under a State system to envisage the alternative situation in which, in order to give them vitality, they are left free to spend Exchequer money without the Minister's approval and to pursue policies which at any rate in detail may not be the Minister's, but for which he would presumably be answerable.

Further, Morrison argued that the Bevan scheme would weaken local government:

It is possible to argue that almost every local government function, taken by itself, could be administered more efficiently in the technical sense under a national system, but if we wish local government to thrive – as a school of political and democratic education as well as a method of administration – we must consider the general effect on local government of each particular proposal. It would be disastrous if we allowed local government to languish by whittling away its most constructive and interesting functions.

In conclusion, Morrison conceded the drawbacks of joint author- ities – 'I dislike them thoroughly' – but urged that while national- isation might be superior to a local authority system 'judged purely as a piece of administrative machinery', this consideration was out- weighed by the political consequences of incurring the antagonism of local government.

So here there is a clear ideological split, not in party terms but in terms of perceived values. On the one hand, there are Morrison's political values: the emphasis on local government as a school of political education, with considerations of efficiency and adminis- trative rationality coming a poor second. On the other hand, there is Bevan's stress on a different set of values: the values of paternal- istic rationalism. For one of the principal justifications advanced by Bevan in his October memorandum to the Cabinet was precisely that nationalisation would be a more efficient and rational system. His scheme, he argued, would enshrine the principle of 'public control following public money'. And it was the only way of achieving 'as nearly as possible a uniform standard of service for all'. As he pointed out, 'Under any local government system – even if it is modified by joint boards or otherwise – there will tend to be a better service in the richer areas, a worse service in the poorer.' So con- siderations of equity reinforced considerations of rationality, and Labour's commitment to equality went hand in hand with argu- ments based on efficiency.

Nor was Bevan prepared to concede that his scheme would pro- duce bureaucratic over-centralisation. 'A centralised service must, indeed, be planned so as to avoid rigidity', he wrote in his counter- blast to Morrison's memorandum',[9] 'that is why I have proposed that the hospital service shall be administered locally by Regional Boards and District Committees. . . . It is precisely by the selection of the right men and women to serve on these bodies that I hope to be able to give them substantial executive powers, subject to a broad financial control, and so prevent rigidity.' But, he conceded that, 'admittedly, this is a field in which there is room for develop- ment in the technique of governments, but the problems that will arise should not be incapable of solution'. Over thirty-five years later the search for new techniques continues, as the problems prove themselves remarkably resistant to the various solutions that have been tried since Bevan wrote his memorandum (see Ch. 3 and 4).

Bevan's view prevailed in Cabinet. But there was a price to be paid; predictably enough, given that any policy choice involved trade-offs between competing considerations. One of the arguments against divorcing control over hospitals from local government was that this would ensure the continued co-ordination, under the same authority, of hospital and personal health services. In his October memorandum Bevan had tentatively, if logically, raised the possibility of transferring responsibility for the personal health services, as well as the hospitals, from local to central government:

the future allocation of the other local government health services – child welfare, district nursing, the provision of health centres for general medical and dental care, and so on – can be considered in detail once a decision in principle has been reached on the hospital services. It looks at first sight as though the ultimate responsibility for these should rest with the Minister, to ensure a unified health service, but there should be provision for delegation to existing persons and agencies for doing the day-to-day job.

However, this suggestion quickly disappeared from view in the subsequent discussions of the legislation: a concession, no doubt, to the Morrisonian advocacy of the local government role. Much of the criticism in the following months, from both the Conservative Opposition and from the medical profession, concentrated precisely on Bevan's failure to achieve a 'unified health service'. Nor was this criticism confined to Bevan's political opponents: one of Labour's backbenchers, Frederick (later Sir Frederick) Messer, argued in the Second Reading debate[20] that Bevan's measure was 'not a health service Bill; it is a medical service Bill'. The divorce between medical services in the strict sense and health services in the wider sense was to become one of the major themes in the continuing debate about the NHS over the coming decades.

Bevan's legislation embodied other concessions as well. There was no concession to the voluntary hospitals as such: unlike local authorities these did not have any spokesmen in the Labour Cabinet, nor did they carry any weight with the Party. But his plans did incorporate some features designed specially to appeal to the most prestigious medical specialists, represented by the Royal Colleges, as part of an overall political strategy of splitting the medical profession. This strategy consisted of buying off the potential opposition of the Royal Colleges, and enlisting their support against the BMA – the voice, essentially, of the general practitioners.

Not only were Teaching Hospitals given special status: with governing bodies of their own directly under the Minister of Health,

The politics of creation

instead of being integrated into the administrative structure of the hospital service. Not only were the regional authorities given executive status, instead of being merely advisory bodies as envisaged in the 1945 proposals of the Conservative Government. But, in addition, the right to private practice in hospital pay beds was enshrined in the legislation, to the dismay of many Labour backbenchers. A new system of merit or distinction awards was also introduced – the brainchild of Lord Moran of the Royal College of Physicians and one of the key actors in Bevan's manoeuvres to enlist the support of the hospital specialists. This was to give consultants deemed to be meritorious by their peers special financial rewards, over and above their basic salaries. Lastly, once the principle of limiting the bodies responsible for the health service to elected local government representatives had been abandoned, the way was open for doctors to serve on the new authorities: something the profession had long fought for, but which the 1944 White Paper had explicitly rejected. 'The full principle of direct public responsibility must, of course, be maintained, but we can – and must – afford to bring the voice of the expert right into direct participation in the planning and running of the service', Bevan wrote in his October memorandum to the Cabinet, introducing his scheme for a National Health Service. As between accountability to elected members and professional participation, the balance had decisively been tilted towards the latter, though in the Second Reading debate Bevan did warn against 'the opposite danger of syndicalism'.

Interestingly, Bevan was not prepared to extend the participation principle conceded to the medical profession to other health service workers. When the Trades Union Congress raised this possibility, Bevan was quick to squash it.[21] No one, he pointed out in a letter to Sir Walter Citrine, the TUC's General Secretary, would be on the Regional Boards and Hospital Management Committees in a representative capacity:

I attach great importance to the principle that these bodies shall consist of members appointed for their individual suitability and experience, and not as representatives or delegates of particular, and possibly conflicting, interests. This means that members of Regional Boards and Management Committees could not be appointed to 'represent' the health workers, and I could not agree to an alternative suggestion that has been put forward – that a proportion of members of these authorities should be appointed after consultation with the health workers. The difficulty here would be to draw any line which would keep membership of the Boards and Committees down to reasonable numbers. If the nurses were to be consulted, why not also the hospital domestics? the radiotherapists? the physiotherapists? and so on.

So while doctors were to participate in the running of the new NHS, representing 'expertise' rather than the medical profession, the same principle was not to be applied to other health service workers: a disparity which was to fuel argument in the 1970s when this issue once again surfaced.

Given these concessions, it is not surprising that the initial opposition to Bevan's proposals for the hospital service soon melted away. Nor, of course, is it surprising that the concessions so made were to become the raw material of future political controversy, in so far as they represented the victory of tactical considerations over administrative and political logic, coherence and consistency. However, it was issues involving general practitioners which aroused the fiercest passions and opposition between 1945 and 1948: so much so, that the ability of the Minister to launch the NHS on the appointed day in July 1948 remained in doubt until almost the last month. Yet, paradoxically, in the case of general practice, Bevan was for the most part content to accept the negotiated compromise that had emerged when he inherited his post.

The single most important feature of Bevan's proposals for general practice was the acceptance of the 1945 Conservative plan for maintaining Insurance Committees in the new incarnation of local Executive Committees (with a stronger representation for the medical profession than under the previous machinery). All doctors would be in contract with this Executive Committee, thus removing any threat of general practitioners becoming either part of a national corps of doctors employed by a Central Medical Board, as envisaged in the 1944 White Paper, or of becoming local authority employees. In this respect, then, Bevan's plan marked a major retreat since 1944, in the face of the medical profession's objections. The medical profession's suspicions were roused by three other aspects of Bevan's proposals. First, it was laid down that Health Centres would be provided by local authorities: this not only fulfilled a longstanding Labour commitment to this kind of practice, but also was designed to serve as a bridge between medical services and the health services provided by local authorities. The change was one more of emphasis than of substance: the 1944 White Paper had stated that Health Centres should be given a 'full trial', while even the Conservative Plan had suggested that there should be a 'controlled trial'. But even this was enough to arouse the latent paranoia of the BMA, which scented the danger of local authority control.

This paranoia was further reinforced by another proposal: this was that general practitioners should be remunerated on the basis of a mixture of part-time salaries and capitation fees. This was not as threatening as the 1944 White Paper, which had proposed full-time salaries for all doctors employed in Health Centres. But it marked a change from the Conservative plan, which had dropped any salaried element. Here the BMA were quick to seize on the thin end-of-the-wedge argument: once even partial salaries were introduced, the way would be open to turn all general practitioners into salaried State bureaucrats. In logic, the BMA was wrong: part-time salaries were in fact introduced in the 1960s (see Ch. 3) without turning general practitioners into salaried officials. In their reading of Bevan's long-term intentions, however, the BMA were right. At a meeting of the Cabinet's Social Services Committee, Bevan said that 'he looked forward towards the establishment of a full-time salaried medical service in due course, but felt that it would be impracticable to make such a major change in established practices at once'.[22] The BMA's ire was further fuelled by the reinstatement of the 1944 White Paper proposal – dropped by the Conservative Government to set up a central Medical Practices Committee which would have the power to prevent doctors from setting up in practice in areas which already had their fair share of medical manpower. Lastly, and this was the only point on which Bevan was more radical than the 1944 White Paper, the Labour Government proposed to prohibit the sale and purchase of practices, and to compensate existing general practitioners accordingly.

It was these proposals which threw a lighted match into the BMA's smouldering discontent. In the long-drawn-out battle that followed, the BMA raised a number of further issues – invariably dressed up in the rhetoric of the threat to the sacred principles of the freedom of patients to choose their own doctors and of the right of doctors to practice their craft free from interference (neither of which were, in fact, threatened by the Labour Government's proposals). The details of the controversy are of little concern here. But two points require noting. First, in April 1948 – when it seemed that the opposition of the BMA would prevent the NHS from getting off the ground on the appointed day – Bevan made what was apparently a dramatic concession. Amending legislation would be introduced to make it clear that it was no part of his intention to create a whole-time, salaried service: general practitioners would continue to be paid on a capitation fee basis – and part-time salaries would be limited to new entrants to the profession for their first three years.

Whether or not this represented a defeat for Bevan is arguable: this depends on just how committed he was to the 'establishment of a full-time medical service', and what he envisaged the timetable of progress towards this policy aim to be – something which cannot be established conclusively on the basis of the available evidence. But the concession was certainly a victory for the medical profession, in that it recognised the principle that it could veto any proposals to change the methods of remuneration: a phenomenon which appears to be international.[23]

Second, the years between 1945 and 1948 help to illuminate the complex nature of intra-medical politics. Indeed the politics of the medical profession, as distinct from the politics of health care, would require a study in their own right to do them anything like justice. The BMA's constitution included, in the words of the Webbs, 'all the devices of advanced democracy'. That is, neither the BMA bureaucracy – led by its Secretary, Charles (later Lord) Hill – nor the elected leadership could commit the Association: all deals had to be referred back to the BMA's representative body. Thus it is not surprising that 25 years later Hill could write, reflecting on that confrontation with Bevan:

It is undeniable that emotional outbursts in public at critical times, inevitable in a large body at times of crisis, did sometimes embarrass the profession's spokesmen by the headlines they stimulated and the somersaults of policy they encouraged. . . . Furthermore, the Representative Body did declare itself – in advance of any Government plans – in favour of many features of a health service which it subsequently rejected. It did tend sometimes to ignore such gains as its representatives had secured and immediately to switch its attention to the points on which it had not won, however important or unimportant they were. Balance sheets of gains and loss are not always judged dispassionately in large assemblies, where oratory and emotion prevail. Tactics are better devised in private by the few than publicly by the many.[24]

This emphasises the danger of 'reifying' the medical profession: to see it as a phalanx of disciplined troops defending clearly defined interests and objectives. The interests of the medical profession were by no means homogeneous: we have already noted the division between the BMA, representing mainly general practitioners, and the Royal Colleges. The objectives, also, differed: as between those who were concerned to promote a technically efficient, high-quality medical service based on consultants and those whose main aim was to conserve a particular way of life based on the GP surgery – between the technicians and the individualists in the profession.

Moreover, on any question of tactics, the profession tended to be split: in the final plebiscite organised by the BMA, to decide the profession's response to Bevan's promise of amending legislation in 1948, 54 per cent were against further discussion with the Minister, while 46 per cent were in favour (with the consultants split evenly, and the general practitioners opposing further negotiations by nearly two to one). Given the constitutional machinery of the profession's organisation, it was always easier to mobilise support for outright opposition rather than to secure agreement on specific proposals – with the consequence that the difficulty in getting agreement on what was or was not acceptable would in turn eventually tend to undermine the commitment to outright opposition. It is, once again, a pattern which provides a *leitmotif* for the history of the NHS: one which helps to explain, for example, the outcome of the protracted negotiations about consultants' contracts in the 1970s (see Ch. 4).

WHOSE VICTORY WAS IT?

So, in July 1948, the National Health Service was launched. It was designed, as Aneurin Bevan told the House of Commons when introducing his Bill, 'to universalise the best': to divorce the ability to get the 'best health advice and treatment' from the ability to pay and 'to provide the people of Great Britain, no matter where they may be, with the same level of service'. It is thus easy to see why the creation of the National Health Service has been seen as a triumph of Socialist ideology, inspired as it appeared to be by egalitarian ideas: a model of institutionalising the principle of allocating resources according to need. From this perspective, if we try to explain the political processes which resulted in the creation of the NHS, there is no need to look further than the election which brought the 1945 Labour Government into power and Bevan into office.

Yet, as the previous account should have made clear, the question of whose victory the creation of the NHS represented allows of no clear-cut answer. For Eckstein,[25] the creation of the NHS represented a victory not so much for Socialist ideology – in the strict sense of being concerned with remedying distributional inequities – as a victory for a 'radically managerial' ideology. Admittedly, the creation of the NHS was part of a long, evolutionary process, in which both the paternalistic rationalists within the civil service and the medical technocrats – the professional elite which sought to maximise the opportunities to deploy the tools of medical science –

played a leading role. From their point of view, the health services as they existed in 1939 presented a policy puzzle: how to make sense of a ramshackle, partly bankrupt, incoherent and incomplete system. As we have seen, much of the process of policy-making represented a series of attempts to test out the 'fit' of various solutions: to reconcile different aims of policy and to minimise opposition. To a large extent, then, the creation of the NHS can be seen as an example of social learning.[26]

Social learning is not, however, a neutral process which takes place in a vacuum of preconceptions and assumptions. What people learn depends on their perceptions of the situation with which they are trying to deal, and the assumptions they bring to bear on problems. The years between 1939 and 1948 show that different actors in the policy machine had very different perceptions and assumptions, and that these differences played a large part in shaping their actions. Thus civil servants tended to put much emphasis on the engineering of consensus, and in particular on avoiding a clash with the medical profession. In this, they were at one with the Conservative politicians. In contrast, Bevan and the Labour Government were prepared to move out of the private arena of health care politics – the engineering of consensus through negotiations in Whitehall – into the public arena of political conflict. The extent of the break with the past, represented by Bevan's arrival at the Ministry of Health, must not be exaggerated: Bevan did not abandon the politics of compromise. If his plans represented a striking innovation in one respect, he largely built on the compromises that had been hammered out over the previous years and paid a heavy price in terms of concessions made to buy off opposition, both from consultants and local government. But there was nothing inevitable about the final shape of the NHS as it emerged in 1948: the same aims of policy could have been achieved through different organisational and institutional means.

Equally, to concentrate on the terms of the debate is to risk missing out on what was, surely, at least as important: those issues which were not debated precisely because all the actors were agreed in their assumptions. If much of the debate was about technical issues – that is, about the appropriate administrative machinery – this was because certain crucial aims of policy were taken for granted. If there was little evidence of Socialist ideology in the debate, if there appeared to be little emphasis on distributional issues, this was at least in part because this was common ground. Nothing is more remarkable than the shared assumption that the health service should be both free and comprehensive – and that it should be based on the principle of the collective provision of services and the pooling of financial risks through the public financing of the service. Even in the years of the Coalition Government, when the Conservatives might have been expected to take a different view, one of the few issues of controversy in the arguments of the Cabinet Reconstruction Committee was the limited question of whether or not there should be hotel charges in hospitals[27] – a question prompted not by ideological considerations but by the practical problem of how best to ensure an independent source of income for voluntary hospitals.

Most important of all, perhaps, the discussions reflected a shared assumption about the past achievements and future potentials of medical science. Implicit in the consensus about the general aims of policy was a shared, optimistic faith in progress through the application of diagnostic and curative techniques. In turn, this mirrored the belief that medical science had not only triumphed over disease and illness in the past but would continue to do so in future. On this view, the only problem was how best to create an institutional framework which would bring the benefits of medical science more efficiently and equitably to the people of Britain. There might be disagreement about specific policy instruments, but there could be little argument about the desired goal or about the eventual rewards.

Again, it is all too easy to present the evolution of policy as though all the sets of actors involved were discrete and homogeneous. This is to miss the flow of ideas across the different categories: to assume that the ideas of, for example, the Socialist Medical Association did not influence the attitudes of the civil servants or the medical technocrats. This is surely to ignore the extent to which all the actors were drawing from a common pool of ideas: the extent to which certain assumptions were important precisely because they had ceased to be controversial and had become part of the conventional wisdom.

If the consensus about the ends of policy has to be stressed, so too has the conflict about means. For it was the question of the means to be used which brought the policy-makers into conflict with the interests that would be affected by the organisational and institutional devices chosen to translate the general aims of policy into practice. The battle was about the instruments of policy: a battle in which the main protagonists were the medical profession. Once more, the question of who 'won' this particular battle allows no simple answer, if only because the medical profession itself was a collection of different (and sometimes conflicting) interests. In the case of general practice, the doctors were in effect conceded a right of veto: a right which they used to maintain the *status quo*. In the case of the hospital services, the NHS was designed to accommodate certain specific interests within the medical profession. But in both cases the power of the medical profession consisted less in being able to impose its will in a positive sense than in being able to block changes. Most important perhaps for the future, the medical profession obtained a monopoly of legitimacy among the health service providers: a unique position, reflected in the participation of doctors in the running of the NHS.

The conflict about means did not, however, simply reflect a clash of interests. It also represented a clash of values. In its final form, as it emerged in 1948, the NHS represented the victory of the values of rationality, efficiency and equity: it was designed to be the instrument of national policies for delivering health care in a rational, efficient and fair way across the country. But as the debates between 1939 and 1948 showed very clearly, there are other values. The case for local government control was based not just on the defence of a particular interest – the existing local authorities – but on a view of the world anchored in the values of localism: a view which stressed responsiveness rather than efficiency, differentiation rather than uniformity, self-government rather than national equity.

Built into the structure of the NHS, therefore, were certain fundamental contradictions. Some of these contradictions reflected political concessions: the deliberate acceptance of imperfections in the grand design in order to minimise opposition. Other contradictions, however, reflected the incompatibility of certain objectives. The history of the NHS since 1948 can largely be seen as the working out of these contradictions: a continuing and never-ending attempt to reconcile what may well turn out to be irreconcilable aims of policy.

REFERENCES

1. MICHAEL FOOT, *Aneurin Bevan*, vol. 2, Davis-Poynter: London, 1973.
2. In many ways, the best account remains, Harry Eckstein, *The English Health Service*, Harvard U.P.: Cambridge, Mass. 1958. At the time of writing, the government documents were not accessible and the book is perhaps biased by the sources that were available: Eckstein's exclusive emphasis on the central role

of the medical profession reflects the fact that the main sources available were the published accounts of negotiations in the medical press. Another account based on published sources is A. J. Willocks, *The Creation of the National Health Service*, Routledge & Kegan Paul: London 1967. The first book to be based on the documents now available in the Public Records Office is John E. Pater, *The Making of the National Health Service*, King Edward's Hospital Fund for London: London 1981. Pater himself was a civil servant at the Ministry during the period in question, and his book therefore is a most authoritative (if extraordinarily discreet and self-effacing) account.

3. POLITICAL AND ECONOMIC PLANNING, *Report on the British Health Services*, PEP: London 1937.

4. BRIAN ABEL-SMITH, *The Hospitals in England and Wales, 1800–1948*, Harvard U.P.: Cambridge, Mass. 1964.

5. MINISTRY OF HEALTH, *Interim Report on the Future Provision of Medical and Allied Services*, HMSO: London 1920, Cmd. 693.

6. ROYAL COMMISSION ON NATIONAL HEALTH INSURANCE, *Report*, HMSO: London 1928, Cmd. 2596.

7. BRITISH MEDICAL ASSOCIATION, *A General Medical Service for the Nation*, BMA: London 1930; Socialist Medical Association, *A Socialized Medical Service*, SMA: London 1933.

8. PUBLIC RECORDS OFFICE, MH 80/24, Minutes of 'The first of a series of office conferences on the development of the Health Services', dated 7 February 1938; Minutes by the Chief Medical Officer, dated 21 Sept. 1939.

9. BENTLEY B. GILBERT, *The Evolution of National Insurance in Great Britain*, Batsford: London 1966.

10. MINISTRY OF HEALTH, *A National Health Service*, HMSO: London 1944, Cmd. 6502.

11. PUBLIC RECORDS OFFICE, CAB 124/244, Memorandum dated 10 Feb. 1944.

12. SIR GEOFFREY VICKERS, *The Art of Judgment*, Chapman & Hall: London 1965.

13. For a detailed study of this issue, see Frank Honigsbaum, *The Division in British Medicine*, Kogan Page: London 1979.

14. PUBLIC RECORDS OFFICE, CAB 87/5, Minutes of the War Cabinet Reconstruction Committee, 10 Jan. 1944 and 11 Jan. 1944. The quotations in the following paragraph also come from the records of these two meetings.

15. PUBLIC RECORDS OFFICE, MH 77/30 A, Draft Cabinet Paper by Minister of Health, June 1945.

16. SIR GEORGE GODBER, *The Health Service: Past, Present and Future*, Athlone Press: London 1975.
17. PUBLIC RECORDS OFFICE, CAB 129/3, Memorandum by the Minister of Health: The Future of the Hospital Services, 5 Oct. 1945.
18. PUBLIC RECORDS OFFICE, CAB 129/3, Memorandum by the Lord President of the Council: The Future of the Hospital Services, 12 Oct. 1945.
19. PUBLIC RECORDS OFFICE, CAB 129/3, Memorandum by the Minister of Health: The Hospital Services, 16 Oct. 1945.
20. HANSARD HOUSE OF COMMONS 5th Series, vol. 422, 30 April 1946. All subsequent quotations from the Second Reading debate refer to this source.
21. PUBLIC RECORDS OFFICE, MH 77/73, Letter dated 18 July 1946.
22. PUBLIC RECORDS OFFICE, CAB 134/697, Minutes of the Cabinet Social Services Committee, 29 Nov. 1945.
23. T. R. MARMOR and D. THOMAS, 'Doctors, politics and pay disputes', *British Journal of Political Science*, 1972, no. 2, pp. 421–2.
24. LORD HILL, 'Aneurin Bevan among the doctors', *British Medical Journal*, 24 Nov. 1973, pp. 468–9.
25. ECKSTEIN *op. cit*, (see ref. 2) pp. 2–3.
26. HUGH HECLO, *Modern Social Politics in Britain and Sweden*, Yale U.P.: New Haven, Conn. 1974.
27. PUBLIC RECORDS OFFICE, CAB 87/5, Minutes of the War Cabinet Reconstruction Committee, 10 Jan. 1944.

Chapter two
THE POLITICS OF CONSOLIDATION

In 1958 the House of Commons held a celebratory debate to mark the tenth anniversary of the creation of the National Health Service.[1] It turned out to be an exercise in mutual self-congratulation as Labour and Conservative speakers competed with each other in taking credit for the achievement of the NHS. Aneurin Bevan proclaimed that the service 'is regarded all over the world as the most civilised achievement of modern Government'. Derek Walker-Smith, the Conservative Minister of Health, produced a statistical litany of success. Since 1949, he pointed out, 'Effective beds are up by $6\frac{1}{2}$ per cent; in-patients admitted are up by $29\frac{1}{2}$ per cent; the ratio of treatment to beds is up by 22 per cent; new out-patients treated are up by 12 per cent, and the waiting lists are down by $11\frac{1}{2}$ per cent'. Diptheria had been conquered; tuberculosis was about to be conquered. 'We have to aim', he concluded lyrically, 'at the prevention and, where possible, the elimination of illness, resulting in a positive improvement in health, reflected in the factory, the foundry and the farm, and not merely in the convalescent home.'

Not all was self-congratulation. Some of the issues which were to emerge more strongly over the following two decades provided an element of dissonance, if in a minor key. Bevan spoke of the poor state of the mental health service: 'Some of our mental hospitals are in a disgraceful condition', he pointed out. Similarly, he touched on the politically sensitive issue of pay beds in hospitals, where consultants could treat their private patients. The system was being abused by some consultants, he claimed, to allow their private patients to jump the waiting list. In turn, Walker-Smith qualified his optimistic vision of progress by conceding that success was creating its own difficulties for the NHS. 'If one is less likely to die of diptheria as a child, or from pneumonia as an adult, one has a greater chance of succumbing later to coronary disease or cancer', he

argued, 'by increasing the expectation of life, we put greater emphasis on the malignant and degenerative diseases which are characteristic of the later years.' An ageing population, and a new pattern of
disease were generating new problems for the NHS.

This anniversary debate provides a convenient, if necessarily
arbitrary, watershed in the political history of the NHS. Ahead lay
the politics of rational planning: a series of endeavours to adapt the
machinery of the NHS in the light of the experience gained and
problems revealed during the first decade. This is the theme of the
next chapter. Behind lay the politics of consolidation: the transformation of what started out as a controversial experiment in social
engineering into a national institution anchored in consensus. This
provides the theme for the present chapter. By 1958 the transformation was indeed complete. 'The National Health Service, with the
exception of recurring spasms about charges, is out of party politics',
wrote Iain Macleod – a former Conservative Minister of Health – in
1958.[2] Some controversies might occasionally disturb the calm of the
political pond: charges was one such issue, pay beds was another.
But as an institution, the NHS ranked next to the monarchy as an
unchallenged landmark in the political landscape of Britain. Public
opinion polls consistently showed a high degree of enthusiasm for
the NHS, with 90 per cent or more of the respondents declaring
themselves to be satisfied with the service. More surprisingly, perhaps, two-thirds of the medical profession declared that – given a
chance to go back ten years and to decide whether or not the NHS
should be started – they would support the creation of the service.[3]

The contrast between this consensus and the political furore that
attended the launching of the NHS is striking. But it is more apparent than real. The rhetoric of battle in the years between 1946 and
1948 served largely to conceal, as we saw in the previous chapter,
the very considerable degree of continuity and compromise involved
in the creation of the NHS. Until Bevan's arrival on the scene, the
norm and style had been closed arena politics: private negotiations
between the various interests within the health care arena. Moreover
Bevan himself, once he had won his victory of principle, quickly
reverted to this style: negotiations about the detailed implementation
of the general principles laid down in the 1946 Act were conducted
in the customary discreet manner between Ministry of Health civil
servants and the representatives of the medical profession.[4] The
depoliticisation of the NHS after 1948 can thus be seen simply as
the re-emergence of organisational routines anchored in the British
tradition of government; in particular, the emphasis on resolving

disagreement by the incorporation of interest groups in the processes of decision-making.[5]

It is, of course, misleading to talk about the depoliticisation of the NHS in a general sense. In the period in question, and indeed later, it was depoliticised only in a very specific sense: that of party politics. The NHS remained a political system in its own right: a political system with its own actors, rules and dynamics. Moreover, even given the absence of party controversy about the fundamentals of the NHS, it was inevitable that the health care system would be influenced by the political environment in which it was operating: the ideological and intellectual assumptions which shaped not only attitudes towards, but also within, the NHS.

This chapter, then, examines the internal politics of the NHS in the decade or so that followed its launching. In doing so, we shall develop some of the themes that emerged in the discussions that led up to the formation of the NHS: to see how the problems and policy dilemmas then identified were, or were not, resolved. But before exploring specific areas we must, however, look at the evolving characteristics of the health care policy arena. Throughout the 1950s, the policy process bore the imprint of three shocks. First, there was the harsh discovery of the gap between the commitments of the NHS and the resources available. Second, there was the gruelling experience of actually getting the NHS off the ground: of putting administrative flesh on the legislative skeleton of 1946. Lastly, the NHS, conceived in an era where the dominant ideology favoured collectivist planning, grew up in an intellectual climate that leant towards minimal government. All three factors helped to shape the assumptive worlds of the policy-makers – their perceptions of what was possible and desirable, what administrative tools could be used – and thus, in turn, influenced the development of the NHS.

INFINITE DEMANDS, FINITE MEANS

In December 1948, only four months after the NHS had been launched, Bevan addressed what was to be the first of a series of self-exculpatory memoranda to his Cabinet colleagues explaining why the service would cost much more than anyone had expected.[6] The original estimate of £176 million for 1948–49 would, he warned his colleagues, turn out to be £225 million:

The rush for spectacles, as for dental treatment, has exceeded all expectations. . . . Part of what has happened has been a natural first flush of the new scheme, with the feeling that everything is free now and it does not matter what is charged up to the Exchequer. But there is also, without doubt, a sheer increase due to people getting things they need but could not afford before, and this the scheme intended.

More important still, he stressed, the cost of salaries and wages had proved much higher than anticipated. He concluded:

The justification of the cost will depend upon how far we get full value for our money; and that in turn will depend on how successfully my Department administers the service, eradicates abuse – whether by professional people or by the public – and is able to control the inevitable tendency to expand in price, which is inherent in so comprehensive and ambitious a scheme as this.

In the event, the Ministry of Health did not appear to be able to 'control the inevitable tendency to expand in price'. A supplementary estimate of £59 million for 1948–49 was followed by one of £98 million for 1949–50. NHS expenditure appeared to be out of control. In 1949 the Government passed legislation giving it power to impose a shilling prescription charge, with the aim both of raising £10 million in revenue and of reducing the 'cascades of medicine pouring down British throats', in Bevan's own phrase.[7] In 1950 Bevan, who despite his public support for prescription charges had fought a private Cabinet battle against their actual introduction, agreed to a compromise whereby a ceiling was imposed on NHS expenditure. Later the same year a special Cabinet Committee, under the chairmanship of the Prime Minister, was set up to 'keep under review the course of expenditure on this Service'.[8] Finally in 1951 the Chancellor of the Exchequer, Hugh Gaitskell, announced charges for dental work and optical service with the aim of containing spending within the £400 million limit set: an announcement which lead to the resignation of Bevan from the Cabinet.

In retrospect, the political furore may seem disproportionate to the cause: a battle fought over paper figures and symbols, rather than real issues. The 1956 report of the Guillebaud Committee, set up in 1952 to inquire into the cost of the NHS, showed that much of the anxiety aroused both by the seeming extravagance of the NHS and by the policy responses had been exaggerated.[9] Much of the apparent increase in spending, it pointed out, was due to general price inflation: 'the rising cost of the Service in real terms during the years 1948 to 1954 was less than people imagined.' Indeed expenditure on the NHS actually fell as a proportion of the national income in the climacteric political year of 1950–51.

As far as charges were concerned, the Guillebaud Committee tended to be agnostic. Charges for dental treatment, the report concluded, had acted as a deterrent and were, in the long run, undesirable; however, given the current shortage of dentists, the Committee thought it would be a mistake to abolish them. Charges for spectacles also acted as a barrier to use, and the Committee recommended that a 'fairly high priority' should be given to a 'substantial reduction' in the level of charges when more resources became available for the NHS. Lastly, the Committee favoured, on balance, the retention of prescription charges (introduced by the Conservative Government in 1952): ' . . . we have no reason to think', the report concluded, 'that the charge hinders the proper use of the Service by at least the great majority of its potential users.' Overall, with some reservations that will be discussed later, the Committee threw out the indictment of extravagance and inefficiency against the NHS: ' . . . allowing for the manifold shortcomings and imperfections inherent in the working of any human institution, we have reached the general conclusion that the Service's record of performance . . . has been one of very real achievement.'

Despite this retrospective vindication, the days of financial innocence for the NHS were over. The original sin of health care utopias – the contrast between infinite opportunities for spending money and all too finite availability of resources – had been revealed. With the benefit of hindsight, this may be an all too obvious point. Yet nothing is more striking in the voluminous files of the discussions that lead up to the creation of the NHS, drawn upon in the previous chapter, than the lack of consideration given to the financial implications of setting up the NHS: even the Treasury dog did not bark. The assumption was that the cost of the NHS could be calculated simply by extrapolating pre-war health care expenditure: hence, of course, the gross under-estimate for the first year of the NHS's operation. No thought appears to have been given to the possibility that a national health service would have a financial dynamic of its own; on the contrary, the assumption was rather that expenditure on health care would tend to be self-liquidating by producing a healthier population. Equally little thought seems to have been given to the income side: the long-term implications of the methods chosen to finance the NHS. It therefore came as all the more of a shock to realise that the logic of the NHS's commitment to providing a free service and to 'universalising the best', in Bevan's phrase, ran counter to the logic of its dependence on the Treasury and tax revenue for funds.

The case for accepting the NHS as an institution which inevitably and rightly generated extra expenditure demands was put by Bevan in a memorandum he wrote for the Cabinet in March 1950.[10]In this he argued that:

Allowing for all sensible administrative measures to prevent waste, the plain fact is that the cost of the health service not only will, but ought to, increase. Most of the hospitals fall far short of any proper standard; accommodation needs to be increased, particularly for tuberculosis and mental health – indeed some of the mental hospitals are very near to a public scandal and we are lucky that they have not so far attracted more limelight and publicity. Throughout the service there are piling up arrears of essential capital work. Also it is in this field, particularly, that constant new development will always be needed to keep pace with research progress (as, recently, in penicillin, streptomycin, cortisone etc.) and to expand essential specialist services, such as hearing aids or ophthalmic services. The position cannot be evaded that a nationally owned and administered hospital service will always involve a very considerable and expanding Exchequer outlay. If that position cannot, for financial reasons, be faced, then the only alternatives (to my mind thoroughly undesirable), are either to give up – in whole or in part – the idea of national responsibility for the hospitals or else to import into the scheme some regular source of revenue such as the recovery of charges from those who use it. I am afraid that it is clear that we cannot have it both ways.

Moreover, there was yet a further reason for expecting the pressure for more NHS expenditure to continue: the demands generated by the professional providers of the service. The whole point of the NHS was, after all, supposedly to eliminate all financial considerations which might inhibit treatment according to need. From the patient's point of view, this meant that there should be no financial barriers at the point of access. From the doctor's point of view, this implied that he should be free to carry out his professional imperative of doing his utmost for the individual patient without regard to the cost. Not surprisingly, therefore, Bevan complained to the Cabinet that: 'the doctors had secured too great a degree of control over hospital management committees, and were pursuing a perfectionist policy without regard to the financial limits which had necessarily to be imposed on this Service as on other public services.'[11] Professional perfectionism, clearly, was not compatible with the public financing of the NHS: a source of stress and tension throughout the history of the NHS – as doctors discovered that a hospital service, which many of them had entered on the presumption that it would free them from all financial inhibitions in the exercise of their craft, had in practice turned them into the State's agents for rationing scarce resources.

The difficulties of containing the rise in costs were compounded by another factor. In the case of the hospital service, the Ministry of Health was in a position to determine total budgets: although, as we have seen, it was not entirely successful in this respect in the first years of the NHS. But hospital service spending accounted for just over half of total NHS expenditure: £229 million out of £367 million in 1950–51. The rest of the expenditure was accounted for by the cost of the general practitioner, pharmaceutical, opthalmic and dental services: drugs alone cost £38.5 million in 1950–51, or over 10 per cent of the total NHS bill. Here the expenditure commitment was – as in the case of the opthalmic and dental services – effectively open-ended. If general practitioners prescribed more, if demand for spectacles or dental treatment increased, then inevitably spending would go up. In this respect, then, governments were on a financial escalator which they could not stop. Charges might be introduced to limit demand; general practitioners might be exhorted to prescribe cheaper, non-proprietory drugs. In the last resort, however, general practitioners were independent contractors. If they decided to prescribe more, or to refer more patients to hospitals for expensive treatment there, there was little that anyone could do. The irony of the NHS as set up in 1948, and perpetuated since, was precisely that it could exercise least control over the gatekeepers to the system as a whole: the general practitioners, through whom all referrals to hospitals were channelled.

Not only had the financial dynamics of creating the NHS been ignored. So had the political dynamics of the system chosen to finance it. By rejecting an insurance-based health service – whose revenue would come from ear-marked contributions – the founders of the NHS ensured that it would have to compete with other government departments for general tax-revenue: with education, housing and all the other claims for resources. If Socialism was the language of priorities, in Bevan's words, it did not follow that the NHS would be at the head of the queue: indeed rival spending ministers collectively might have an incentive to squeeze the share of the NHS in the total public expenditure budget (though they might also have a collective interest in maximising the total spent). Even if the public were well disposed towards the NHS, it did not follow that they would cheerfully accept higher taxes to pay for it, since there could be no direct relationship between higher spending on the NHS and higher taxation – given that all the revenue went into the general Treasury fund.

The reasons for rejecting an insurance-based system of finance were expounded by Bevan in the tenth anniversary debate. First, there were considerations of equity. The nature of the treatment given should not have to depend on the contributions made: 'We cannot perform a second-class operation on a patient if he is not quite paid up.' Second, the aim was to make the financial basis of the NHS redistributive. By drawing on general taxation, the system would ensure that those who had the most would pay the most: 'What more pleasure can a millionaire have than to know that his taxes will help the sick?' 'The redistributive aspect of the scheme was one which attracted me almost as much as the therapeutical', Bevan concluded in his retrospective reflections (although even the assumption that general taxation must necessarily and inevitably be progressive is questionable: in practice, the distributive impact depends on variable political decisions about the level and structure of taxes).

The outcome of the decision to reject an insurance-based finance was that the NHS at this period, and subsequently, was financed overwhelmingly out of general tax revenue. In 1950–51, 88.3 per cent of its income came from this source – a proportion which has fluctuated over the years but never fallen below 77 per cent.[12] Health insurance contributions were not dropped – what Treasury would ever agree to abandon a money raising device once it had been introduced? – but became a sort of vestigial financial appendix: once the insurance principle had been scrapped, they were merely another means of raising what was in effect tax revenue. In 1950–51 they accounted for 9.4 per cent of the NHS's total income, a proportion which rose to 17.2 per cent in the early 1960s but subsequently declined to something approaching the original figure.

Another way of raising revenue for the NHS was, as we have already noted, to impose charges on users. The attraction of this was, and remains, that it allows the NHS to generate income in a way which is not competitive with other departments: in theory, it provides a magic formula for raising the spending-power of the NHS while not increasing public expenditure – pleasing both the advocates of higher health spending and the Treasury. In the event, however, charges have never contributed more than marginally to the NHS's income, even though the Conservative Government which came into office in 1951 did not share Labour's ideological

commitment to the principle of a free health service and soon introduced prescription charges. In 1950–51, revenue from this source
was less than one per cent of the NHS's total budget and reached
only 5.3 per cent at its peak in the 1950s.

The reasons were simple and, although the controversy about
charges continued to simmer away throughout the history of the
NHS, were fully explored in an exchange of notes between Bevan
and the Treasury in 1950.[13] If charges were more than nominal,
there would have to be ways of exempting the least well-off. Any
system of exemptions would mean, Bevan argued, 'administrative
complexities and costs', as well as bringing back the means test into
the health service. Equally, exemptions would reduce the total yield.
Even a hotel charge of ten shillings a week for hospital patients,
Bevan pointed out in response to Cabinet pressure, would yield a
total revenue of only £10 million. It is precisely this balance between
high administrative costs and relatively low yields which helps to
explain why hotel charges – which were to be considered by subsequent Conservative Governments almost as a matter of routine –
have never been introduced: an example of ideology yielding to
administrative expediency. Indeed the reconciliation of ideological
considerations and financial necessity was to depend on administrative ingenuity and innovation: the Labour Government of the 1960s
managed to reconcile itself to prescription charges by introducing
an automatic system of exemptions for certain broad categories –
such as the young and the old – so avoiding both the costs and the
political stigma of the means test. But, as always, there was a trade-
off: administrative simplicity meant a lower income, since 60 per
cent of prescriptions fell into the exempt category. There was no
magic formula, as it turned out, for solving the NHS's financial
dilemma.

The nature of this dilemma was clear by the beginning of the
1950s. On the one hand, there were the collective, environmental
pressures to restrain expenditure: an alliance of Cabinet Ministers
and taxpayers, as it were. On the other hand, there were the ever-
present, institutionalised pressures for higher spending. As the Guillebaud Committee pointed out: 'It is still sometimes assumed that
the Health Service can and should be self-limiting, in the sense that
its own contribution to national health will limit the demands upon
it to a volume that can be fully met. This, at least for the present,
is an illusion.' There was no way of setting a financial target, the
report further commented, which would ensure that an 'adequate
service' would be provided: 'There is no stability in the concept

itself: what might have been held to be adequate twenty years ago would no longer be so regarded today, while today's standards will in turn become out of date in the future. The advance of medical knowledge continually places new demands on the Service, and the standards expected by the public also continue to rise.'

Politicians, in short, had invented a financial treadmill for themselves when they created the NHS: whatever their political investment in raising funds, they would be chasing a metaphysical, ever-elusive concept of adequacy. They could never do enough. The NHS was a machine for generating new demands: a point recognised in Walker-Smith's tenth anniversary speech quoted at the beginning of this chapter. It is therefore scarcely surprising that in the 1950s the NHS evolved from being an instrument for meeting needs (as conceived by the founding fathers) to becoming an institutional device for rationing scarce resources.

There is another aspect of the debates about NHS finance which requires stressing. This is the language used. Bevan, as we have seen, fully accepted the existence of 'abuse' in the use of services. Moreover, he had talked about the 'cascades of medicine' pouring down British throats. It was imperative, everyone agreed, to stop waste and extravagance. In short, by the beginning of the 1950s, the NHS was stereotyped as a spendthrift organisation: a service which, moreover, had exploited its lack of financial control to grab more scarce public resources than those government departments which had actually managed to keep within their budgetary allocations. From the point of view of the Treasury, vice had been rewarded in the 1940s, and the 1950s were marked by a determination not to allow history to repeat itself. In the assumptive world of the Whitehall policy-makers, the NHS remained for most of the decade an undeserving case.

Not surprisingly, therefore, the NHS had to live on short-commons for most of the 1950s although this was a decade of booming economic growth by British standards at least. In 1958, its income (in cost terms, at 1970 prices) was only three per cent higher than it had been in 1950, while expenditure on education had soared.[14] Moreover, as the Guillebaud Committee pointed out, it had been starved of money for capital investment: its capital investment programme was running at a much lower level than that, even, of the pre-war hospital system. In turn, this slow rate of growth – and the perception of the NHS as a penitent financial sinner – affected the policy-makers both at the Ministry of Health and at the periphery: the subject of the next section.

WHATEVER IS BEST ADMINISTERED IS BEST

In the 1940s, the Ministry of Health was a department which was breaking exciting new ground. In the 1950s, it was the department which had to be stopped from doing things: in particular, as we have seen, from spending money. So it is not surprising that, if the years leading up to 1948 represent a case study in the politics of innovation, the decade that follows represents a case study in the politics of exhaustion. The emphasis switched from political to administrative decisions: from maximising the opportunities for change to minimising the dangers of turbulence. In a very real sense, the 1950s thus represent a breathing space between the crisis of creation in the 1940s and the renewed interest in change that characterised the 1960s. They are a period in which the stress was on achieving organisational stability: financially the new NHS had shown a cloven hoof, and now the emphasis was on seeking respectability.

In forging this new style, three sets of actors were involved: the politicians, the civil servants and the NHS administrators. Perhaps a fourth set of actors should also be considered: the medical profession. Their role is analysed in a subsequent section. Here we concentrate on the first three sets of actors. All had rather different interests and ideologies. However, in the 1950s – though not always subsequently – they shared, if for different reasons, the same quietist orientation. Taking first the political actors, the most important factor was also the most obvious one: in October 1951, a Conservative Government was voted into office. It had been elected on the slogan of 'Set the people free'. The thrust of Tory policy was to disengage from intervention in the workings of the economy. The remnants of wartime controls were scrapped; the process of nationalisation was reversed. The rhetoric of free market economics replaced that of national planning. Although the existence of the NHS was not threatened, it was operating in a different ideological and intellectual climate from that of the 1940s: from being the favourite child prodigy of the Government, it had become the somewhat embarrassing legacy of a previous liaison between Labour politicians and over-enthusiastic planners.

Whether as a direct consequence or not, the status of the Ministry of Health diminished. The process had already begun under the Labour Government. Following Bevan's translation to the Ministry of Labour in January 1951, the department's local government functions were grafted onto the new Ministry of Local Government and Planning. Its staff was, at a stroke, cut from 5,300 to 2,724: from being one of the most impressive mansions in Whitehall, it had become a semi-detached villa. At the same time, the Ministry lost representation in the Cabinet: a status it did not regain until its fusion with the Ministry of National Insurance under Richard Crossman in the late 1960s. But the process of decline in status accelerated under the Conservative Government when the Ministry became something of a revolving door for politicians. For the ambitious career politicians, it was only a resting place on the way to higher things. For others, it became a consolation prize on the way to backbench oblivion. Between 1951 and 1958, there were no less than six different occupants of the ministerial post.[15]

Of these Iain Macleod, Minister of Health from 1952 to 1955, was the outstanding figure. Not only did he stay longer than anyone else in the 1950s: more than three years. He was also the only political heavyweight: a future Conservative Prime Minister that was never to be. It is therefore all the more significant that he saw his role at the Ministry as one of consolidation, not innovation. Within a fortnight of arriving at the department, he told his officials that he wanted the health service to enjoy a period of tranquillity, with no drastic reorganisation.[16] Too much legislation had been passed, and too many instructions had been issued, he argued in a speech in 1952: 'It is about time we stopped issuing paper and made the instructions work. I want to try and recreate local interest and above everything to get a complete partnership between voluntary effort and the State.' The encouragement of voluntary work became one of Macleod's main themes, just as it became the theme of another Conservative Minister – Patrick Jenkin – at the end of the 1970s: again a period of financial stringency for the health service, when invoking voluntary effort could be seen as a way of overcoming the inadequacies of public finance (and also a period when an ideology of minimal government was dominant).

Macleod's recessive style at the Ministry of Health accurately mirrored the prevailing mood of the Government as a whole. In turn, if for somewhat different reasons, his approach chimed well with the administrative biases of the department in the 1950s. Its senior officials – lead by Sir John Hawton, Permanent Secretary from 1951 to 1960 – were veterans of the battles of the 1940s and the subsequent investment of effort in getting the NHS off the ground. 'After 1948', one of them remarked, 'a great many people felt that they had as much change as they could take.' It was perhaps not surprising that the shell-shocked survivors of encounters with the medical profession in the 1940s – who decades later could still remember the angry representatives of the doctors pounding the table with their fists at meetings and shouting in unison – did not want to risk repeating the experience. Moreover, the strain had been carried by a very small number of officials. In 1951, the Ministry still only had 21 men and women above the principal rank, backed by 48 principals and assistant principals. Nor did this handful of civil servants engaged in policy work have much in the way of support. It was not until 1955 that the Ministry appointed its first statistician; the Guillebaud Committee recommended, with some asperity, the creation of a statistical and research department. Qualitatively, too, the Ministry of Health was perhaps lacking, though here the evidence is at best tentative. Among successful candidates for the administrative civil service, it came low in the pecking order.[17] In the view of one BMA participant in negotiations with the Ministry, the department 'became the dumping ground for third-rate civil servants': an example, possibly, of how the Whitehall perceptions of a department as being something of a backwater, whose main achievements lie in the past, may become self-reinforcing.

Above all, though, there had been the sheer administrative slog of getting the NHS off the ground. The NHS, as conceived in the 1946 legislation, was hardly more than an outline sketch. It is only in trying to grasp the sheer enormity of the administrative task involved in the late 1940s that it is possible to understand the department's style and stance in the subsequent decade. For the Ministry of Health, the creation of the NHS involved the setting up of a new administrative structure and devising a new set of rules and regulations for making it work. The members of the new authorities had to be selected. A new machinery of negotiation, for dealing with the 55 professional associations or trade unions that represented the NHS's workers had to be set up: the Whitley Council system which brought together the spokesmen of the employees and the employers. Regulations, embodying conditions and terms of work had to be negotiated not only with the medical profession but with a 'bewildering variety of professional societies, covering workers as diverse as chemists and chiropodists, matrons and midwives, physicists and pharmacists, radiographers and remedial gymnasts.'[18] A vast range of administrative questions, concerned with the detailed delivery of the NHS's services, had to be hammered out in consultation with the representatives of the medical profession. Just taking the year 1948–49, these included such issues as the fees to be paid to general practitioners for vaccinations and immunisation, the lay-out of the Health Service prescription book, the supply of pessaries and Dutch caps, mileage allowances for rural practitioners and problems regarding certificates to enable patients to obtain surgical corsets.[19] All this was in addition to the ever-interesting, all-absorbing topic of levels of pay, about which more in a following section.

To set out this agenda for action, if only selectively, is not only to underline the burden involved. It is also to indicate the technical nature of many of the issues involved. In turn, the special nature of decision-making at the Ministry of Health was reflected in the departmental structure. Parallel to the civil service hierarchy culminating in the Permanent Secretary there was a professional hierarchy culminating in the Chief Medical Officer (CMO): the voice of expertise within the department. Like his lay counterpart, the Chief Medical Officer had direct access to the Minister (although one Permanent Secretary described the relationship between himself and the CMO as follows: 'We walk through the corridor arm-in-arm, but when we come to a door, I go through first').

From the point of view of the medical administrators, the problem of running the NHS was essentially that of concerting the activities of the consultants and general practioners, all of whom were intensely individualistic and all of whom saw themselves as accountable only to their professional peers. From this perspective, the role of a central government department could only be to prompt and to encourage the evolution of medical practice: 'You help professional opinion to form itself spontaneously', as one experienced medical administrator put it. The point is well caught in the following quotation from Sir George Godber, who was CMO from 1960 to 1973 and a dominating figure in the first thirty years of the NHS:

The NHS is comprised of very many services rendered daily by physicians, nurses, dentists, pharmacists and others. The content of those services is defined, not by planners, but by essential professional knowledge and skills. Change in method and practice is brought about by intra-professional exchanges; it may be abrupt because of a scientific development such as the advent of a new drug, or it may occur gradually with experience.[20]

Policy change can thus only be an adaptive process: 'there is no initial revelation from an all-wise centre', but a gradual process of professional consensus-building. Central government might use expert committees of professionals to push along the process, but it could not instruct or command.

The emphasis in the 1950s on keeping the machinery running, on care and maintenance rather than innovation and change, also reflected the interests and ideology of our third set of actors in the health policy area: the administrators of the NHS. At the periphery, too, the creation of the NHS involved a heroic administrative undertaking. New administrative authorities – 14 Regional Hospital Boards (RHBs), 36 Boards of Governors for Teaching Hospitals and some 380 Hospital Management Committees (HMCs) – had to be set up. Staff had to be recruited: one new RHB started life with only a couple of clerks.[21] Information had to be collected: the new staff often did not know the hospitals in their area and lacked even basic data about the number and distribution of doctors within their administrative fief. Once appointed, the officers had to work out their style of administration. This was not easy. At every level of the NHS there were three hierarchies of officers. There were the lay administrators: descendants of the pre-NHS hospital secretaries. There were the medical administrators; and there were the finance officers. In principle, the relationship was one of equality of status, but in practice the early years of the NHS were often marked by fierce battles between the three categories of officers. In some authorities, the lay administrators sought to establish their primacy over the treasurers: the case is quoted of one Finance Officer not being allowed to see his daily post until it had been opened and perused by the Secretary. In other instances, the Senior Administrative Medical Officer sought to impose his primacy as against the lay administrator.[22] In no case, however, was there a simple administrative hierarchy incorporating all the disciplines.

From the start, too, the NHS's administrative structure had a characteristic which helped to shape the relationship between centre and periphery throughout its existence. This was that all officers were appointed and employed by individual authorities, whether RHBs or HMCs. Although there were national conditions of pay and service, there was nothing remotely resembling a national corps of administrators or even a national policy for recruitment and training. The values and traditions of localism were thus built into the administrative structure of the NHS from the start. Not only were most of the original staff recruited from local government or the voluntary hospitals, where the tradition had been that of loyalty to a specific authority or to a particular institution. But they also became, in their new incarnation, the servants of individual NHS authorities, sharply distinguished from the civil servants of the Ministry of Health. There was no convergence in the career paths of NHS administrators – whether lay, medical or financial – and those of the central government civil servants. If an NHS administrator wished to enhance his reputation, he would do so not by demonstrating his ability to carry out national policies, but by showing his capacity for running the affairs of his own parish smoothly and effectively. In effect, his constituency was local, not national: his occupational incentives were thus biased towards accommodating local pressures rather than implementing central government exhortations, should there be any conflict between the two.

So much for the specific political biases, administrative styles and problems of implementation in the first decade of the NHS. But, before turning to a discussion of specific policy issues that surfaced in the 1950s, it is essential also to identify some of the more general characteristics of the arena of health care policy which constrained policy-makers not only in the 1950s but subsequently as well. First, to make explicit what so far has been implicit, the NHS is an institution marked by its complexity and its heterogeneity. The NHS is complex in that its workings depend on the spontaneous interaction of a large variety of different groups with different skills, all dependent on each other: from doctors to nurses, from laboratory technicians to ward orderlies (a complexity which has increased over the years with increased occupational specialisation). It is heterogeneous in that it delivers a wide range of different services under the same organisational umbrella: from acute care to chronic care, from maternity services to mental handicap services. In both these respects, other public services – education, for example – are relatively simple administrative organisms in comparison with the NHS.[23] In both these respects, too, the NHS presents special problems which affect both policy-making and administration.

Second, compounding the problems of policy-making, the health care policy arena is characterised by the ambiguity of objectives and uncertainty about the means needed to achieve any given ends. The point about ambiguity of objectives can be simply illustrated. From one perspective, increasing patient throughput can be seen as a measure of success in terms of improving productivity and treating illness; from another perspective, though, it may be seen as an indicator of failure to prevent disease. Similarly, there is frequent uncertainty about how best to achieve any given end: what level, or mix, of skills and resources is required to provide a particular kind of service. Moreover, given the ambiguity of objectives and uncertainty about means, there are no generally acceptable measures of performance which would allow the success or failure of the NHS to be assessed. In a sense, the output of the NHS *is* the organisation. It is this which explains one of the dominant features of the assumptive world of policy-makers in the 1950s and later: dominant precisely because unargued. This is the dependence on professional judgements – that is, the judgement, primarily though not exclusively, of the medical profession – on issues of need and adequacy. Lacking independent criteria of their own, policy-makers were forced to fall back on the professional view of what services were needed and how quality should be assessed. In a sense, this dependence can in part also be seen as a legacy of the assumptions which went into the building of the NHS, discussed in the previous chapter: specifically, the assumption of the paternalistic rationalisers that the objective of a health service should be to create a world fit for experts to apply their skills to the entire population. But it was reinforced in the 1950s by political consensus which left the way clear for problems and issues to be defined within the health care arena through the perceptual lenses of the professionals.

It is against this background that we have to explore the specific policy issues that emerged in the 1950s. In what follows, this chapter will examine three policy themes which allow us to examine the way in which the problems and dilemmas inherent in the creation of the NHS worked themselves out in this period. First, what balance was struck between central and local autonomy? Second, what progress was made towards Bevan's objective of 'as nearly as possible a uniform standard of service for all'? Third, what were the consequences of institutionalising the 'voice of the expert' – that of the medical profession – in the structure of the NHS? In each case, the aim is not to provide a history of events but to analyse the dynamics of the policy process.

CENTRE-PERIPHERY RELATIONS: THE CIRCLE REFUSES TO BE SQUARED

In setting up the NHS the aim was to reconcile national accountability and local autonomy. Public control had, inevitably, to follow public money: the Minister of Health was accountable to Parliament for every penny spent in the NHS. In turn, Members of Parliament could and did ask questions both about broad issues of policy or expenditure and about the detailed delivery of services. In 1950, MPs asked 629 questions; in 1955, they asked 1,045.[24] The Public Accounts and Estimates Committees of the House of Commons examined, in detail, the way in which the NHS spent public money. Yet at the same time the dangers of bureaucratic over-centralisation had to be avoided: the RHBs and the HMCs had to be given, in Bevan's words, 'substantial executive powers'.

It is therefore not surprising to find, throughout the first decade of the NHS, two contrasting themes running through the debate about relations between the central government department and the peripheral health authorities. From the centre came pressure on the Ministry of Health to exercise stricter control over what was happening at the periphery.[25] Rumbling through successive reports of the Public Accounts and Estimates Committees are demands for stricter central control in the pursuit of national uniformity: demands which were, of course, fuelled by the sense of NHS expenditure being out of control. From the periphery, however, there came complaints that the Ministry of Health was interfering too much: drowning administrators in a stream of circulars. Already in March 1948, even before the NHS had formally been set up, the chairmen of the RHBs were protesting that the Ministry was not letting them get on with their job by meddling in the affairs of HMCs.[26]

The Ministry of Health's dilemma can best be illustrated by the problem posed by the challenge of bringing expenditure under control. In 1950 Bevan appointed a senior civil servant with wide experience in other departments, Sir Cyril Jones, to study the financial workings of the NHS.[27] In his report, Jones identified what he saw to be the 'fundamental incompatibility between central control and local autonomy'. This stemmed, as he saw it, from the separation of the responsibility for raising and for spending money:

The old compulsions in favour of financial responsibility in hospital administration have now disappeared, viz. the limit of private generosity in the case of voluntary hospitals, whose greatest assets when appealing for public support were long waiting lists and bank overdrafts; and the odium of raising rate revenue in the case of the local authority hospitals. Something is needed to take their place if the situation is not to get completely out of hand, now that hospitals are administered by voluntary workers who, keen and public spirited though they be, bear no responsibility for providing the funds and cannot be called to account by those who have to pay the bill. The only sanction is the ultimate drastic step of dismissal which, if once invoked, would practically kill voluntary service in this field.

Moreover, Jones pointed out, the difficulties for the Ministry of Health were compounded by lack of information:

The fact is that the Ministry possesses very limited information regarding the financial administration of the hospitals of the country on the basis of which . . . the estimates are framed; has no costing yardsticks at its disposal by which to judge the relative efficiency or extravagance of administration of various hospitals, and hence no alternative but either to accept the estimates wholesale as submitted without amendment, or to apply overall cuts to the total budgets in a more or less indiscriminate manner.

The Jones report has been quoted for the insights it provides into the centre–periphery relationship in the early years of the NHS. His recommendations for action were, however, largely ignored. Chief among these was one which was to crop up again and again during the following thirty years but never to be implemented: this was the abolition of the regional tier of administration. RHBs, Jones argued, 'should cease to be directly concerned with hospital administration and become regional hospital planning bodies'. HMCs, in turn, should become 'subject to direct control by the Ministry', to be exercised through a system of out-posting Ministry civil servants.

A number of other recommendations which came to nothing are also worth nothing. First, Jones directly challenged 'the doctor's right to prescribe for his patient, as he wishes'. In the case of more expensive appliances, Jones thought, such decisions should be reviewed by the lay managers of the service. Second, Jones argued for the exclusion of doctors from the management authorities of the NHS: 'in any democratic organisation it is axiomatic that, while due regard must be paid to the advice of the technical experts, if there is the slightest suspicion that such experts may have a direct or indirect pecuniary or other self-interest in any matters, they should not be parties to the making of decisions thereof.' In any case, there was 'no reason in principle for according hospital medical staffs a privileged position as compared with that of other members of the hospital staff'.

The medicine was too strong for Bevan: a reminder that radical politicians may, in practice, be more conservative than civil servants who do not carry the political costs of implementing change. From Bevan's point of view, the costs of changes which threatened the position of the medical profession would be too great: 'Frankly, I do not consider the battle worthwhile.' While in principle he accepted the idea of relegating the RHBs to an advisory role, yet he was sceptical of giving the Ministry greater direct responsibilities:

There would have been no theoretical difficulty – there is none now – in having from the outset a tightly administered centralised service with all that would mean in the way of rigid uniformity, bureaucratic machinery and 'red tape'. But that was not the policy which we adopted when framing our legislation. While we are now – and rightly, I think – tightening up some of the elements in our system of financial control, we must remember that in framing the whole service we did deliberately come down in favour of a maximum of decentralisation to local bodies, a minimum of itemised central approval, and the exercise of financial control through global budgets, relying for economy not so much on a tight and detailed Departmental grip, but on the education of the bodies concerned by the development of comparative costing, central supply and similar gradual methods of introducing efficiency and order among the heterogeneous mass of units we took over.

In the outcome, the financial crisis of the late 1940s and early 1950s did lead to one basic change. What had started out as a bottom-up system of generating budgets – with demands coming from the local hospital authorities – became a top-down system of dividing out a fixed total: of determining capped budgets for individual authorities.[28] In effect, the dilemma of central control *v.* local autonomy was, in the case of expenditure, side-stepped by allowing a very large degree of discretion *within* the centrally sanctioned budgetary limits. The 'exercise of financial control through global budgets', in Bevan's words, became the guiding principle of the NHS.

Briefly, the panic about overspending did lead to more direct Ministry intervention at the periphery. In 1950 the Ministry sent out teams of experts to review the staffing establishment of hospital authorities; the exercise was designed particularly to cut administrative staff. But the lapse into interventionism was brief. From 1952 onward, responsibility for control over establishment was transferred to the RHBs. When in 1951 the Ministry launched yet another economy drive, the emphasis was on local responsibility for implementing national policy: the department underlined the 'scope for local initiative in discovering and stopping extravagance and waste'. The concept of this exercise – 'a review inspired and stimulated from the centre, but devised and applied locally'[29] – was to become the model of Ministry policy-making throughout the 1950s, and indeed much later.

Overall it is possible to see an evolving philosophy of administration in all this: a philosophy of administration which saw policy as the product of interaction, rather than as the imposition of national plans.[30] The centre provided the financial framework and advice about desirable objectives. It left the periphery free to work out the details: rationality, from this perspective, lay in recognising that the complexity and heterogeneity of the NHS made it impossible to impose uniform national standards from the centre. Nothing more was heard in the 1950s about the 'rational and effective' plans for local health services envisaged in the 1944 White Paper. The acceptance of diversity, in short, was not only a necessary concession to the principle of localism but an inevitable outcome given the nature of the NHS. The centre, quite simply, did not know best – and indeed could not know best. There was a further ingredient, however, in this philosophy of administration. Even when the centre did know best – even if governments did have clear views about what was desirable – it did not perceive itself to be in a position to command. It could educate, it could inspire and it could stimulate. To have done more would have run counter to the values both of localism and of professionalism. It would have undermined the autonomy of health authorities and challenged the right of professionals to decide the content of their work.

It is this which explains what is perhaps the hallmark of Ministry of Health policy-making in the 1950s: policy-making through exhortation.[31] Circulars poured out of the Ministry: an average of about 120 a year in the 1950s. Some half of these had to do with the implementation of Whitley Council decisions: that is, the national decisions about conditions and terms of pay and service. Others were more technical in nature: requests for information, guidance about building standards. There was also a core of circulars which gave advice about desirable patterns or standards of service provision. To the extent that these affected the practices of the professionals, however, these could only be hortatory – given the acceptance of the principle of professional autonomy. This principle of professional autonomy did not only apply to the doctors. It applied equally to other professionals, such as nurses. Thus, to take the example of an issue which has continued to be a subject of controversy throughout the history of the NHS, in 1949 the Ministry of Health asked hospital authorities to make it easier for parents to visit their children in hospital. Three years later, however, an inquiry into actual practices showed that only 300 out of the 1,300 hospitals admitting children were allowing daily visiting, while about 150 did not allow any visiting at all.[32] Those responsible for local decision-making – in this instance, primarily the nurses – had chosen largely to ignore the centre's advice.

Although, therefore, there continued to be a tension between national accountability and local autonomy throughout the 1950s – and subsequently – the balance had swung towards the latter. The local health authorities were seen not so much as agents of the Ministers but as independent bodies. 'The Minister seeks to act always by moral suasion', a departmental civil servant told the Estimates Committee. The paradox of financial stringency was that while it led to tighter control over the total budgets available to health authorities, it also weakened the centre's ability to use incentives to persuade the periphery to follow national policies: the Ministry of Health could neither command nor bribe.

THE PATTERN OF INEQUALITIES

Financial stringency had one further perverse effect. The problem of 'perpetuating a better service in the richer areas, a worse service in the poorer' – which Bevan had seen as the main argument against a local government based health service – was, in the outcome, perpetuated in the 1950s. The inherited inequalities in the geographical distribution of hospital beds – a useful though only partial indicator of the distribution of resources generally – remained virtually undisturbed. For example, in 1950 Sheffield RHB had 9.4 beds per 1,000 population, while the South-West Metropolitan RHB had 15.1. Ten years later, the equivalent figures were respectively 9.1 and 14.2.

In effect, under the pressure of financial crisis and in the absence of the information needed to make judgements about local services and needs, the Ministry of Health settled in the 1950s for control over the inherited budgets of local health authorities as distinct from trying to devise what would be an appropriate financial allocation from first principles. Primacy was given to the issue of control, to the neglect of the issue of distribution. 'The criticism is still made, however, that the system favours most the authorities who showed the least degree of financial responsibility in the early years of the service', the Guillebaud report noted, adding, 'We agree that the main weakness of the present system of allocating revenue funds is the lack of a consistent long-term objective.' Given the overall constraints on the total NHS budget, this outcome was perhaps inevitable. The lack of substantial growth in the total budget meant that any policy designed to improve the geographical distribution of resources would, in fact, have had to be a policy of re-distribution: of actually taking funds away from the best endowed parts of the country to transfer them to the least well-equipped regions. At a time when the overriding aim of policy was to achieve stability and to avoid turbulence, this was unlikely to be appealing. In any case, given the pressures of pent-up demands everywhere, even the best off regions had no difficulty in making out a case for the inadequacy of their existing allocations. So, not surprisingly, the principle of basing allocations on historical inheritances – of giving priority to maintaining the existing service – triumphed.

In theory, the capital budget could be used to infuse new resources into the relatively deprived regions of the country: as the

Guillebaud Committee noted, five per cent of the total national sum available for capital spending was reserved for the 'seven Hospital Regions needing special help'. But as the capital investment programme never topped £50 million (at 1970 prices) in the 1950s, this five per cent hardly represented a crock of gold. In any case, immediate need was the enemy of long-term planning: as one Ministry of Health civil servant saw it, 'From the beginning we gave priority to the worst off areas. But as soon as you did this, you came up against the problem of the London Teaching Hospitals. They were all falling down. Do you let them fall down? Or do you give more resources to London, which is already well stocked?' In the event, the decision was to shore up the existing buildings: symbolic perhaps of health policy generally in the 1950s.

The success or otherwise of improving the distribution of NHS resources cannot, of course, be measured in terms of the numbers of beds alone. This is, at best, only a very partial measure of access to health care. Equally important is the distribution of skilled medical manpower. In the case of general practitioner services, the NHS – as we saw in the previous chapter – introduced a system of negative controls, designed to prevent general practitioners from entering practice in the relatively well-endowed parts of the country: a policy which succeeded in reducing the proportion of patients in under-doctored areas, those where the list sizes were exceptionally large, from 51.5 per cent in 1952 to 18.6 per cent in 1958.[33] In the case of hospital consultants, however, new policies had to be devised. The history of these policies provides an illuminating case study: an example both of the rational planning precepts of the pre-NHS days being carried into effect and of their subsequent dilution under the pressure of financial, professional and administrative constraints.

In the field of specialist services, the NHS started out with two aims in 1948. The first was to increase the availability of such services by creating more consultant posts. The second was to improve their distribution, both geographically and as between different specialties. To meet both objectives, the Ministry produced in 1948 what was in effect a national plan for the specialist services.[34] This set out what was considered to be an appropriate norm of consultant posts, by different specialties, for any given population. But hardly had the circular left the Ministry than the NHS was struck by financial crisis. The expansion of the consultant posts slowed down and the targets receded into the indefinite future. Subsequently, in 1953, an Advisory Committee on Consultant Establishments was set up: a medical committee acting as agent for the Ministry. Its function was to consider all applications for the creation of new consultant posts. As in the case of general practitioners, the policy instrument for improving the distribution of consultants was negative in character. 'The committee simply advised on applications received; it could not seek them out from regions thought to be in greatest need', was the subsequent comment of Sir George Godber, the author of the 1948 plan.[35] Implicitly the hopes of introducing national standards for medical manpower had been abandoned: given financial stringency, the emphasis was on rationing rather than planning.

Overall, the creation of the NHS did increase access to specialist services. The number of consultants rose from 5,316 in 1949 to 7,031 in 1959, although as late as 1962 nearly all the specialties were below the targets proposed in the 1948 circular. A higher proportion of the increased total was, moreover, in precisely those areas of medicine which had failed to attract specialists in the pre-NHS days: for example, anaesthetics and psychiatry. So, with qualifications, this can be seen as a success story for the NHS. However, it once again illustrates the way in which the initiative passed from the centre to the periphery during the 1950s: with central government reacting to demands coming from the medical profession and the peripheral health authorities, rather than shaping the pattern of the service being provided.

PROFESSIONAL INFLUENCE AND PUBLIC POWER

In giving an account of the role of the medical profession in the NHS during the 1950s, it is possible to present two contradictory but entirely accurate conclusions. On the one hand, it is possible to demonstrate convincingly that the NHS exploited its position as a virtual monopoly employer of medical labour to depress the incomes of doctors. On the other hand, it is possible to show equally convincingly that the medical profession permeated the decision-making machinery of the NHS at every level and achieved an effective right of veto over the policy agenda.

'The unnerving discovery every Minister of Health makes at or near the outset of his term of office is that the only subject he is ever destined to discuss with the medical profession is money', wrote Enoch Powell, in his reflections on his own period in office.[36] Indeed the politicisation of conflict over money is inherent in the nature of the NHS. Given that the NHS has a virtual monopoly of employment of medical manpower, there is no independent market for determining the appropriate income for doctors. The Ministry of

Health not only determines the demand for medical manpower but also the supply (through its decisions about the appropriate number of medical school places). It is therefore not surprising that the 1950s – like subsequent decades – were marked by a series of conflicts over pay between the medical profession and the Ministry of Health, and a succession of attempts to devise a neutral machinery of arbitration. Thus the first decade of the NHS was punctuated both by regular confrontations between the medical profession and the NHS over pay and by equally regular references to neutral arbitrators. In the 1940s, the Spens Committee sought to establish a pattern of pay derived from the pre-war incomes of doctors. In 1951, Mr Justice Danckwerts adjudicated on the vexed question of how to adjust the Spens recommendations in the light of the changing value of money. In 1957, a Royal Commission on Doctors' and Dentists' Remuneration[37] was set up to examine levels of remuneration and to examine ways of regularly reviewing pay.

The report of the Royal Commission is significant for the evidence it provides of how the medical profession had fared financially during the first decade of the NHS. In the event, the Royal Commission tended to substantiate the grievances of the doctors. 'At the time of our appointment current earnings of doctors and dentists were too low', the Commission concluded. Further, it pointed out, medical salaries had continued to fall behind earnings in comparable professional occupations. General practitioners had done particularly badly. Between 1950 and 1959, the average person in Britain had become almost 20 per cent better off in real terms, while the average general practitioner had become about 20 per cent worse off. The Royal Commission not only recommended all-round increases. It also recommended the creation of a permanent review body which would regularly inquire into medical pay, mainly though not exclusively using the comparability criterion to ensure that doctors kept in line with men and women in other professions (such as accountancy and the law) where there was no government monopoly of employment.

If the power of any interest group is to be measured by its ability to secure resources for its own members, the medical profession must thus be rated as a failure in the 1950s. If the doctors saw themselves as the exploited victims of the NHS system, they were largely right. Moreover, in this respect, they did no better – or worse – than other employees of the NHS. For example, the salaries of health service administrators also fell, in real terms, by something like 20 per cent during the 1950s.[38] What this would suggest is that the power of the medical profession is in an inverse relationship to the size of the stage on which a specific health care issue is fought out. When the stage widens to bring on actors who normally play no part in the health care arena strictly defined – when the Treasury and the Cabinet become involved – then the ability of the medical profession to get its own way diminishes.[39] Once the issue is defined as that of financial control – when it is seen, in other words, as an issue revolving round national economic strategy rather than health care considerations – the medical profession simply becomes a small battalion facing heavyweight armies. Conversely, the medical profession's influence expands as the stage narrows: becoming in effect total when health care reaches the stage of a duet between doctor and patient.

The point can be illustrated by the instance of general practitioner pay. This, in the 1950s, was based on the 'pool' system. That is, a given amount of money was set aside as the pool from which all payments would be made to general practitioners: in effect, very much the same kind of 'capped' budget which was introduced for hospital authorities. The Ministry of Health's main concern thus was to contain the total size of the pool; an endeavour in which it was remarkably successful, as the earnings figures already cited indicate. However, once control over the total had been established, the Ministry was quite prepared to make concessions to the BMA about the detailed way in which capitation fees and other elements were calculated. Here the story is that of a series of concessions to the doctors.

In discussing the role, influence and power of the medical profession (or indeed of any other professional body or interest group), it is thus crucial to specify the limits of the arena in which the question is being asked. If one is prepared to draw those limits tightly enough – to put the spotlight on an area of concern so small as to be of interest only to a particular profession or interest group – then it is easy enough to conclude that the power of that profession or interest group is dominant. Thus if one were to study NHS policy on methods for making beds, then inevitably the conclusion would follow that the power of the nursing profession is absolute. What distinguished the medical profession in the 1950s, however, was the extent to which it permeated the institutional decision-making machinery of the NHS as a whole. Once an issue had been defined to belong to the health care arena (as distinct from the wider political stage), it was the doctor who represented the voice of expertise. In the mid-

1950s, the Guillebaud Committee noted, the medical membership
of RHBs averaged 32 per cent: in one case it reached 42 per cent.
In the case of HMCs, the proportion tended to be somewhere
between 20 and 27 per cent. Similarly, the Executive Committees
– responsible for general practice, among other services – had a statutory minimum of 4 medical representatives out of a total membership of between 20 and 40.

The Guillebaud Committee saw no objection in principle to medical membership, although it thought that the total should not go
above 25 per cent. The inclusion of doctors, it argued, provided
'invaluable advice to the lay members on medical aspects of hospital
management'. Of course, this is to beg the question of how to define
the 'medical aspects'. Indeed it is tempting to argue that the real
political battle in the health care arena is precisely a definitional one:
whether or not specific problems or issues should be labelled as
being essentially 'medical' in nature, and as such taboo for the non-
expert. Clearly, the institutionalised medical voice within NHS
authority provided doctors with an opportunity to medicalise management: to define issues in terms which would ensure that they
would represent legitimate, expert authorities. In addition, these
authorities were, in turn, festooned with medical advisory committees, placed at every tier of the management structure.

In summary, then, the power of the medical profession – if one
may be allowed to use that slippery concept – rested on two pillars
in the 1950s. First, there was its ability to determine which issues
were or were not put on the agenda for action: certain policy options,
as we saw in the previous section, were ruled out of court because
the political costs of confronting the medical profession were judged
to be excessive. Second, the medical profession to a large extent succeeded in defining certain areas as out of bounds to non-profession-
als: its power lay, as it were, in shaping the perceptions of policy
problems – of incorporating a professional bias into the assumptive
worlds of the policy-makers. While it did not dominate the NHS in
terms of getting what it wanted in a positive sense, it did succeed
in asserting its right of veto in specific policy spheres. Above all, the
medical profession had made sure that governments, whatever their
ideology or ambitions, would think long and hard before seeking to
change the structure of the NHS in any way which would bring the
underlying concordat with the medical profession into question:
from being the main opponents of the NHS, the doctors had in effect
become the strongest force for the *status quo*.

The politics of the National Health Service

AGENDA FOR THE FUTURE

The 1950s bequeathed a long agenda for action to the next generation of NHS policy-makers. Some of the unresolved issues have been discussed in the preceding pages. Others, however, were also clamouring for attention. Above all, there were the problems of co-ordination stemming from the division of responsibility as between the hospital, the general practitioner and the local authority services. Britain, as yet, only had a national hospital service. Could this be translated into a national health service? The question perturbed the Guillebaud Committee which decided, however, that stability must come first: the shock of creation had not yet worn off, and it was premature to think of any radical reorganisation. Equally, the question perturbed nearly everyone who considered the practical problems of the NHS: the Central Health Services Council – charged with producing reports on general policy issues – gave much thought to the obstacles to co-operation between the hospital, local authority and practitioner services.[40]

The triumph of the 1950s was to make the NHS work: but the price paid for creating a consensus – for putting the emphasis on achieving financial respectability, administrative stability and professional acceptability – was to introduce a bias towards inertia. The first decade of the NHS may not have solved the policy dilemmas inherent in the creation of the NHS, discussed in the previous chapter. But it made them tolerable; furthermore, it created a powerful constituency for the *status quo*. Thus, ironically, one of the measures of the success of the first generation of NHS policy-makers was the difficulty faced by their successors in creating a new consensus and mobilising a new coalition for change, as the politics of consolidation gave way to the politics of movement: the theme of the next chapter.

REFERENCES

1. HOUSE OF COMMONS HANSARD 5th series, vol. 529, 30 July 1958.
2. IAIN MACLEOD ET. AL, *The Future of the Welfare State*, Conservative Political Centre: London 1958.
3. The data about public and medical opinion is taken from surveys conducted by Gallup Polls. I am grateful to Gallup Polls for allowing me access to their archives.
4. HARRY ECKSTEIN, *Pressure Group Politics*, Allen & Unwin: London 1960.

5. For a discussion of corporate bias in the British system of government, see Keith Middlemas, *Politics in Industrial Society*, André Deutsch: London 1979.
6. PUBLIC RECORDS OFFICE, CAB 129/131, The National Health Service: Memorandum by the Minister of Health, 13 Dec. 1948.
7. Quoted in Philip M. Williams, *Hugh Gaitskell*, Jonathan Cape: London 1979. For accounts of the battle between Bevan and Gaitskell over charges from the point of view of the two protagonists, see this and Michael Foot, *Aneurin Bevan, 1945–1960*, Davis-Poynter: London 1973.
8. PUBLIC RECORDS OFFICE, CAB 134/518, Cabinet Committee on the National Health Service: Composition and Terms of Reference, Note by the Prime Minister, 22 April 1950.
9. COMMITTEE OF ENQUIRY INTO THE COST OF THE NATIONAL HEALTH SERVICE, *Report*, HMSO: London 1956, Cmnd. 663. The statistical work, on which the Committee based their conclusions, was carried out by B. Abel-Smith and R. M. Titmuss; see their *The Cost of the National Health Service in England and Wales*, Cambridge U. P. 1956.
10. PUBLIC RECORDS OFFICE, CAB 129/38, National Health Service: Control of Expenditure, Memorandum by the Minister of Health, 10 March 1950.
11. PUBLIC RECORDS OFFICE, CAB 128/17, p. 104.
12. All historical statistics about NHS expenditure and income are drawn from Tables E6 to E11 in: Royal Commission on the National Health Service, *Report*, HMSO: London 1979, Cmnd. 7615. Being on a constant price basis (at 1970 prices) these are not directly comparable with figures of actual spending – as given, for example, in the Guillebaud Committee.
13. PUBLIC RECORDS OFFICE, CAB 129/39, National Health Service: Memorandum by the Minister of Health, 30 March 1950.
14. For comparative statistics of public expenditure on different programmes, see Rudolf Klein, 'The Politics of Public Expenditure: American Theory and British Practice', *British Journal of Political Science*, Oct. 1976, pp. 401–3.
15. For the record, the Ministers were: H. Marquand (Jan.–Oct. 1951); H. Crookshank (Oct. 1951–May 1952); I. Macleod (May 1952–Dec. 1955); R. Turton (Dec. 1955–Jan. 1957); D. Vosper (Jan. 1957–Sept. 1957); D. Walker-Smith (Sept. 1957 –July 1960).
16. This account of Macleod's ministerial career is drawn from: Nigel Fisher, *Iain Macleod*, André Deutsch: London 1973.

The politics of the National Health Service

17. MAURICE KOGAN, 'Social Services: Their Whitehall Status', *New Society*, 21 August 1969.
18. ALEC SPOOR, *White-collar Union: 60 Years of NALGO*, Cox & Wyman: London 1967.
19. ECKSTEIN, *op. cit.*
20. SIR GEORGE GODBER, 'Decision-making System and Structure in the British National Health Service', *Hospital Progress*, vol. 57, no. 3, 1976.
21. SIR GEORGE GODBER, *The Health Service: Past, Present and Future*, Athlone Press: London 1975.
22. CHRISTOPHER HAM, *Policy-making in the National Health Service*, Macmillan: London 1981.
23. RUDOLF KLEIN, 'Costs and Benefits of Complexity: the British National Health Service' in Richard Rose (ed.), *Challenge to Governance*, SAGE Research Series in European Politics vol. 1, Sage: London April 1980.
24. I am grateful to Dr Renuka Rajkumar for carrying out this laborious analysis.
25. By far the best study of administration in the NHS in the 1950s is the Acton Society Trust study of *Hospitals and the State*, London 1955. In what follows I draw heavily on this.
26. PUBLIC RECORDS OFFICE, MH 90/54, Chairmen of Regional Hospital Boards: Note of Meeting held on 16 March 1948 at the Ministry of Health.
27. PUBLIC RECORDS OFFICE, CAB 134/518, Cabinet Committee on the National Health Service: Enquiry into the Financial Working of the Service – Report by Sir Cyril Jones. The comments by Bevan, quoted subsequently, form an introduction to this report.
28. For a description of the system of budgeting, see Ministry of Health, *Report for the Year Ending December 1952*, HMSO: London 1953, Cmd. 8933.
29. *Ibid.*
30. For a recent analysis of alternative styles of policy-making, see C. E. Lindblom and D. K. Cohen, *Usable Knowledge*, Yale U. P.: New Haven, Conn. 1979.
31. J. A. G. GRIFFITH, *Central Departments and Local Authorities*, Allen & Unwin: London 1966.
32. MINISTRY OF HEALTH, *op. cit.*
33. The discussion of medical manpower draws on Rosemary Stevens, *Medical Practice in Modern England*, Yale U. P.: New

Haven 1966. The discussion of consultant policy also draws on this invaluable source.

34. The circular in question was RHB (48)1; its author was the future Chief Medical Officer, Sir George Godber.
35. SIR GEORGE GODBER, *Change in Medicine*, Nuffield Provincial Hospitals Trust: London 1975.
36. J. ENOCH POWELL, *Medicine in Politics*, Pitman Medical: London 1966.
37. ROYAL COMMISSION ON DOCTORS' AND DENTISTS' REMUNERATION, *Report*, HMSO: London 1960, Cmnd. 939.
38. SPOOR, *op. cit.*
39. This conclusion reflects the argument of Eckstein, *op. cit.*
40. CENTRAL HEALTH SERVICES COUNCIL, *Report on Co-operation Between Hospital, Local Authority and General Practitioner Service*, HMSO: London 1952.

Chapter three

THE POLITICS OF TECHNOCRATIC CHANGE

If the first decade of the NHS was the period of consolidation, the next decade and a half was the period of innovation. The financial sinner had done penitence; the years of sackcloth and ashes were over, and a new era of expansion began. The politics of administering the *status quo* gave way to the politics of technocratic change. At long last the paternalistic rationalisers – those who, in the years before 1946, had seen the creation of a national health service as an opportunity to apply expert knowledge to dealing with need in a planned and systematic way – came into their own.

The shift in perceptions, style and policies was both made possible and constrained by political consensus. The NHS emerged from its first decade, as noted in the previous chapter, as a national monument. Both the main political parties were in agreement about its underlying philosophy and basic structure: an agreement that only started to get frayed towards the end of the 1970s. Overarching consensus about essentials did not, of course, rule out political skirmishes about specific issues. The Labour Party regularly raised the issue of medical charges in election campaigns rather like a mediaeval army carrying the embalmed body of a saint into battle; there were, as we shall see, other areas of disagreement. But given the continuing evidence of the popularity of the NHS – confirmed by every public opinion poll – there was no incentive to challenge the prevailing consensus. On the contrary, the NHS provides a case study of the politics of competition, as against the politics of confrontation: with both the main parties competing to establish their claim to be considered the NHS's best friend. In 1959, for example, the Conservative Party manifesto promised a 'big programme of hospital building', the development of local authority health and welfare services and a major programme to promote good health: 'We shall not only clear the slums, but also wage war on smog . . . and tackle the pollution of rivers and estuaries.' The Labour manifesto countered by pointing out that 'the Tories have completed only one new hospital', and promising that 'as a minimum we shall spend £50 million a year on hospital development'. In addition, it pledged itself to creating an occupational health service, to developing the family doctor service 'and to safeguarding the health, welfare and safety of people employed in shops and offices'. Finally, it promised to abolish all charges.[1]

In 1964, again, the language was that of rival salesmen. The Conservatives proclaimed that their hospital plan would ensure that 'every man, woman and child in the country has access to the best treatment'. It pointed out that: 'We aim to build or rebuild 300 hospitals of which over 80 are already in progress.' Community services would expand: the 'crucial work of the family doctor' would be encouraged; the law controlling the safety and quality of drugs would be improved and: 'We shall also continue our campaign against the enemies of good health, by eliminating slum environments, reducing air pollution and cleaning the rivers and beaches.' Conversely, the Labour manifesto claimed that the NHS 'has been starved of resources', and promised to remedy this situation. The 'inadequate' Tory hospital-building programme would be reviewed and given the necessary finance. The number of qualified medical staff would be greatly increased, more resources would be devoted to research and a 'new impetus' would be given to the development of community care services. It also, of course, promised 'to restore as rapidly as possible a free Health Service'. Charges apart, there is no sign here of political disagreement about policy aims: only about which party would provide the appropriate level of financial resources.

When party politics end, administrative technology comes into its own. If it is possible to characterise the health care policy arena from about 1960 to 1975 (the dates are to an extent arbitrary) as being about the politics of technocratic change, it is because the debate was about instruments rather than ideologies, about means rather than about ends. Consensus in the era of non-growth had meant making the best of the *status quo*. Consensus in an era of growth meant an opportunity to develop new policy tools and organisational formulas: to let the experts loose on the problems that had had to be put into cold storage during the lean years. However, consensus also imposed constraints. It meant that new policy tools and organisational fixes had to be developed in such a way as not to threaten the implicit concordat – particularly with the medical profession – that underlay the creation of the NHS. It set a boundary to the concepts of the feasible used by policy-makers: it strictly defined the limits of the possible within which change could be considered. To have crossed these boundaries, to have broken through the limits, would have risked the re-politicisation of health, and that no party wanted.

There is yet a further reason why the 1960s and the first half of the 1970s can be interpreted as the heyday of technocratic politics in the NHS. It is the emphasis on efficiency and rationality in the use of resources which marked this period. A concern about efficiency was not, of course, unique to this period. There were efficiency drives in the early 1950s, just as there were efficiency campaigns in the late 1970s. But what marks out the period in between is the development of an ideology of efficiency: the idea that policy should be directed towards squeezing the greatest possible output of health care – that elusive concept – out of an inevitably limited input of resources. Already in 1959 the Ministry of Health had set up an Advisory Committee for Management Efficiency; expenditure on 'hospital efficiency studies' rose from £18,000 in 1963–64 to £250,000 in 1966–67.[2] Economists, who did not exist as far as the Ministry of Health was concerned in the 1950s, had by the 1970s established themselves in the department as the twentieth-century equivalents of the domestic chaplains – keepers of the faith of efficiency. The translation of this ideology into practice was slow, halting and incomplete, as we shall see, but the permeation of its concepts and vocabulary into the policy debate helped to shape both the way in which problems were defined and the solutions that were considered.

In all this, the arena of health care policy accurately reflected changes in the wider political environment. The emphasis on achieving greater efficiency and rationality through planning – through the use of new techniques of government – was common to both main political parties: not for the first time did the search for national efficiency spill over into the sphere of social policy.[3] Harold Macmillan, the Conservative Prime Minister from 1957 to 1964, had earlier in his career written a book expounding the case for 'economic efficiency and rational social organisation': an aim which was to be achieved by having more planning and less competition.[4] In the early 1960s, his Chancellor of the Exchequer set up the National Economic Development Council, which introduced indicative planning to Britain.[5] In 1965, the Labour Government of Harold Wilson which had taken office the previous year, published its National

Plowden report
1961

plan[6] based on the assumption not only that economic growth could be planned but also that planning would in turn promote growth. In 1970 one of the first actions of the Conservative administration of Edward Heath was to publish a White Paper on the reorganisation of central government[7]: the aim was to improve the 'efficiency of government', in part by strengthening the analytic capacity of the administrative machine.

New techniques of government were developed. A new machinery for controlling public expenditure – the Public Expenditure Survey Committee (PESC) system – was set up in 1961.[8] Its origins lay in the Plowden report,[9] published in the same year, which can be read as the manifesto of technocratic rationalism in government. The aim of public expenditure control, the Plowden report argued, should be to achieve stable long-term planning: 'chopping and changing in Government expenditure policy is frustrating to efficiency and economy.' There would have to be greater emphasis on the 'wider application of mathematical techniques, statistics and accountancy': for example, the Plowden report pointed out, such techniques might permit 'improvements in the method of making allocations of funds between the Regional Hospital Boards'. In turn, such a system could lead to more explicit choices and debate about priorities.

Three aspects of this new administrative rationalism, shared by both civil servants and politicians, should be noted. First, there was the faith in techniques: such as cost–benefit analysis, PPB (Planning, Programming, Budgeting) and PAR (Programme Analysis Review). Second, there was the belief that to change organisations could improve policy outputs: the 1960s saw a succession of committees charged with the reform of the civil service and local government. Third, organisational reform was largely seen in terms of giving a greater role to expertise. For example, the 1968 report of the Fulton Committee on the Civil Service[10] was much concerned with devising ways of producing a more professional corps of administrators – more managerial, more numerate and more specialised than the traditional generalist. Similarly, the 1969 report of the Redcliffe-Maud Royal Commission on Local Government was preoccupied with the problem of devising authorities large enough to employ a 'wide variety of qualified staff'.[11] All three themes – the emphasis on techniques, on organisational fixes and on creating a machinery of administration designed to give scope to experts – find an echo in the health care policy arena.

Putting a date on the introduction of this new ideology of rationality is, of course, essentially arbitrary. The start of a more expansionist and interventionist era certainly precedes 1960: perhaps the most significant symbolic event in the evolution of government policy was Macmillan's decision in 1957 to allow his Chancellor of the Exchequer to resign rather than to cut public expenditure. In the health care policy arena, 1960 can sensibly be taken as the beginning of a new era. In that year, both the political and the administrative direction of the Ministry changed. The new Minister was Enoch Powell; the new Permanent Secretary was Sir Bruce Fraser; and the new Chief Medical Officer was Sir George Godber. Quite apart from their individual qualities, the appointment of these three was important for what they represented. The arrival of Enoch Powell marked the end of the Ministry of Health as a political backwater. Idiosyncratic, and destined to end in the political wilderness, he could not however be described as a political lightweight. His immediate successor was a future Conservative Chancellor of the Exchequer, Anthony Barber; while the amalgamation of the Ministries of Health and National Insurance into the new conglomerate Department of Health and Social Security in 1968 ensured Cabinet status for the office holder. The appointment of Sir Bruce Fraser meant that the Ministry was no longer headed by an administrator scarred by the experience of setting up the NHS. Fraser's appointment not only gave the Ministry of Health a stronger voice within Whitehall – he had previously been Third Secretary at the Treasury; it also brought into the Ministry some of the notions about long-term expenditure planning that, as already noted, were stirring within the Treasury and were enbodied in the PESC system. Lastly, the promotion of Sir George Godber brought to the top of the medical hierarchy within the Ministry someone strongly committed to the ideas that had originally inspired the creation of the NHS. A radical egalitarian, the author of the 1948 plan for a rational, uniform distribution of medical specialists, he had never lost sight of Bevan's hope of universalising the best.

So the 1960s open with new men in the arena of health care policy acting in a new political environment: an essentially optimistic and expansionary environment, strong in the conviction that government action could promote economic growth. In the sections that follow, we shall examine the confrontation between new attitudes and old problems in specific policy areas. But first, as essential background to understanding the way in which individual policy issues were defined and addressed, we shall explore the apparent paradox of a growing awareness of scarcity of resources in a period of expansion.

GROWING SCARCITY IN AN ERA OF GROWTH

The fifteen years from 1960 to the mid-1970s were a period of rapid growth in public expenditure.[12] While for most of the 1950s, public spending had only slowly crept up, from 1960 onward the growth rate accelerated: a trend maintained under both Labour and Conservative governments. The NHS was one of the main beneficiaries of this trend. Between 1950 and 1958, its current budget increased by only 12.8 per cent in volume terms – that is, the input of real resources. But between 1958 and 1968, the equivalent increase was over 26 per cent. Between 1968 and 1978, the rise was almost as large again.[13] Moreover, expenditure on the NHS increased throughout these two decades proportionately faster than the growth in the national income: the NHS's share of the Gross Domestic Product rose from 3.5 to 5.6 per cent. Significantly, the growth rate of the NHS budget was not related to the political complexion of the government. Indeed, contrary to what might perhaps be expected, the NHS budget grew fastest under the 1970–74 Conservative administration; in contrast, the growth rate was marginally slower under the 1964–70 Labour Government, compelled by economic crisis to renege on its commitment to accelerate the growth of the Welfare State.

So why did increasing affluence lead to an ever more emphatic realisation of the inadequacy of the available resources and to an ever greater stress on efficiency? To answer this question it is necessary to identify the pressures and constraints faced by policy-makers during this period. Not all of them were by any means unique to this period; on the contrary, many of them simply represented a more explicit recognition of problems that had always been implicit in the structure of the NHS. In examining the debates of the 1960s and 1970s we shall often catch echoes of issues already discussed in the previous chapter. But even if many of the problems and dilemmas were in no sense novel, there is a new sharpness in the way they were perceived: they had reached the stage of what – to adapt Stendhal[14] – might be called *crystallisation* in the policy process.

One elegant explanation for the apparent paradox of financial stringency in a period of expansion was provided by Enoch Powell in his reflections on his period of office as Minister of Health, already quoted in the previous chapter[15]:

There is virtually no limit to the amount of medical care an individual is capable of absorbing [Further,] not only is the range of treatable conditions huge and rapidly growing. There is also a vast range of quality in the treatment of these conditions . . . There is hardly a type of condition from the most trivial to the gravest which is not susceptible of alternative treatments under conditions affording a wide range of skill, care, comfort, privacy, efficiency, and so on [Finally,] there is the multiplier effect of successful medical treatment. Improvement in expectation of survival results in lives that demand further medical care. The poorer (medically speaking) the quality of the lives preserved by advancing medical science, the more intense are the demands they continue to make. In short, the appetite for medical treatment *vient en mangeant*.

New advances in medical science, or drug therapy, might help to eradicate some diseases. In the late 1940s and early 1950s, tuberculosis was a case in point – though the relative contribution of drug therapy and improved social conditions is disputed.[16] In the 1960s, there was the hope that drug therapy would permit mental hospitals to be closed down: a hope which, however, still awaits fulfilment. But new techniques were creating new demands. In the 1960s, for example, there was the development of renal dialysis. In the 1970s, there was the development of plastic hip replacement surgery. Both advances in technology were self-evidently socially desirable: renal dialysis saved lives, while hip replacement surgery made life much more tolerable for those otherwise crippled by arthritic conditions. Nevertheless, they helped to reinforce the sense of the NHS at the mercy of the technological imperative: driven by forces over which it had no control – though we shall examine below some of the attempts to contain the demands generated by the extension of the realm of the possible in medical intervention.

Then, again, there was the ageing population. In 1951 there were just under seven million men and women over the retirement age. In 1961 the equivalent figure was 7,700,000. In 1971 it had topped nine million. Moreover, within these rising totals, the proportion of over-75s was also increasing: precisely those people most likely to require health care. To the technological push, there had to be added the demographic pull. Simply coping with the changing population structure, it was reckoned, would require an extra one per cent annual increment in health spending. No wonder, then, that there was growing concern with efficiency: not only in the use of resources by the NHS, but in the way the health service was organised – given that the care of the elderly, in particular, spanned the hospital, general practitioner and local welfare services.

Lastly, although it makes sense to talk about the closed arena of health politics during the period covered by this chapter, the characteristics of the actors involved were changing. In the 1950s, as previously noted, the medical profession and other NHS exployees did relatively badly in terms of income compared to the rest of the population. In the 1960s and 1970s, this began to change. One set of statistics tells the story: that of the relative price effect – which measures movements in the costs of inputs to the NHS (mainly wages and salaries) compared to movements in costs in the economy as a whole. In the 1950s, the relative price effect was negative: the NHS was buying its inputs of manpower more cheaply than other employers. Thus between 1950 and 1958, as we have seen, the volume of inputs into the NHS went up by 12.8 per cent. But the cost of those inputs went up by only 2.9 per cent. Between 1958 and 1968, however, the reverse was true. The cost of inputs rose faster than their volume: that is, the relative price effect turned against the NHS – a trend which was to continue in the 1970s.

In turn, this reflects a new mood of militancy among those working in the NHS. Denied the opportunity to exit from a service with a near-monopoly of employment for health care professionals, they engaged in voice[17] in the NHS, i.e. the politics of protest. In the case of the medical profession, as we shall see, there was increased conflict *among* doctors: general practitioners challenged the differentials between themselves and consultants, junior hospital doctors challenged the differentials between themselves and consultants, while in turn consultants rebelled against the erosion of the differentials between themselves and the rest of the profession. The established professional bodies – notably the BMA – faced increasing competition from rival groups; so undermining still further the notion of the medical profession as a monolithic entity, as it splintered into different and opposed interest groups. Others working in the NHS – organised in both professional bodies and trade unions – also became assertive. From being an oasis of industrial peace, the NHS became relatively dispute-prone. While in 1966 only two stoppages were recorded in the NHS (and an average of 0.69 days lost per 1,000 staff, as against the national figure of 100 days lost per 1,000 employees), in 1973, 18 stoppages were notched up as a result of a national strike by ancillary workers (and an average of 117.8 days lost as against a national figure of 1,104 days lost).[18] So increasingly, in the period in question, the NHS can be conceived of as a machine for generating demands, not only for more resources but also for higher rewards for the service producers.

Moreover, awareness of the perverse financial incentives built into the very conception of the NHS became sharper during the 1960s. Again, this was already implicit in the very early days of the

NHS.[19] However, the 1960s are marked by the development of an intellectual debate which made these issues explicit and gradually introduced them into the language of politics. In particular the debate sharply defined the issue: was the problem one of constraining the demands made by consumers of health care or of restraining the demand generated by the producers of health care? Depending on the definition of the problem, different solutions would follow. On the one hand, the theorists of the private market argued that individuals as consumers of health services would always demand more services privately than they would supply publicly as taxpayers.[20] Given a free service with no price constraints, it was argued, there was every incentive for consumers to make unlimited demands: it was irrational to restrain demands. Yet equally, as taxpayers, they had every incentive to minimise their contribution. The solution therefore was to invoke the price mechanism: to move from State finance to private finance. On the other hand, however, it could be argued that consumer demand in effect controls itself. Even if consumers did not pay cash for medical attention, they incurred time-costs: rationing through queueing in the surgery and the waiting list. It was the producers – the doctors – who generated demands: indirectly by shaping the expectations of consumers, directly by their decisions as to what resources to apply to the treatment of any given patient.[21] From this perspective, the dilemma of policy was not how to restrain consumer demands through the price mechanism but how to reconcile the professional imperative of doctors to maximise the treatment given to any one patient with the need to maximise the health of the population at large: between an absolutist ethic of treatment and a utilitarian approach to resource use.[22] Given an absolutist ethic, it followed that every patient had to be given the best possible treatment: that the limits of treatment should be defined not by resource availability but by the current state of medical knowledge. Given a utilitarian approach, it followed that the criteria of treatment should be determined by the need to maximise the health of the population, not by the need to do everything possible for the individual patient. Indeed, following this line of reasoning, it might well be appropriate for patients to get less than optimal treatment as defined by the medical profession.

Growing awareness of the implications of financial stringency thus brought out into the open a conflict between the two main sets of actors in the health care policy arena: a conflict reflecting different values and perceptions of the aims of a health service. This was the conflict between the professional providers and the paternalistic rationalisers: between the medical profession and the policy nexus of Ministers and civil servants. Oversimplifying, the conflict was between those who saw the aim of the health service as being to provide doctors with sufficient resources to pursue the professional imperative of maximising treatment for the individual patient and those who saw the aim of the health service as being to distribute inevitably scarce funds in such a way as to reconcile the competing claims of different groups for resources. 'The doctor is primarily involved with the individual, the politician inevitably predominantly with groups of individuals', wrote Dr David Owen, a Minister of Health in the 1970s.[23]

If the underlying conflict could not be wished away, could it be eased by devising ways of raising more money for the NHS? Not surprisingly, this question came increasingly to be debated in the 1960s and 1970s. Predictably, given our analysis, the medical profession became increasingly vociferous in its demands for expanding the NHS budget. In 1967, a leading medical figure wrote[24]:

It is the clear duty of the medical profession to present to Government and public the grim and sober truth, that without a vast increase in national expenditure on the hospitals, here and now – and far beyond anything so far envisaged even on paper and for an indefinitely receding future – they will progressively run down, and the present inadequate service will shortly give place to one that is frankly third-rate.

The same year the BMA set up a panel to look into the finances of the NHS which, in due course, came out in favour of an insurance-based system.[25]

Politicians were also preoccupied by the same question. In 1967 Douglas Houghton, Chairman of the Parliamentary Labour Party and previouly the Cabinet Minister responsible for co-ordinating the social services, wrote: 'It can be contended that, judged from the standpoint of the quality and efficiency and adequacy of the services, we are now getting the worst of both worlds. The government cannot find the money out of taxation and the citizen is not allowed to pay it out of his own pocket.'[26] He proposed raising more revenue through charging. In 1969 Richard Crossman, by now Secretary of State for Social Services, gave an equally pessimistic diagnosis, not so very different from that made earlier by Enoch Powell:

The pressure of demography, the pressure of technology, the pressure of democratic equalisation, will always together be sufficient to make the standard of social services regarded as essential to a civilised community far more expensive than that community can afford. It is a complete delusion to believe that if we had no further balance of payments difficulties social service Ministers would be able to relax and assume that a kindly Chancellor will let each one of them have all the money he wants to expand his service. The trouble is that there is no foreseeable limit on the social services which the nation can reasonably require except the limit that the Government imposes.[27]

In contrast to Houghton, Crossman rejected the policy option of charging more. In part this may have reflected his awareness of the political sensitivity of the issue: a sensitivity sharpened by the experience of the Labour Government which had abolished pre-scription charges on coming into office in 1964, only to reintroduce them four years later when economic crisis compelled the Cabinet to choose between cutting NHS spending and finding new sources of income. 'The party meeting on prescription charges was the worst we have ever had', Crossman recorded in his diary.[28] Moreover, the decision to give automatic exemption from charges to broad cate-gories of the population – like the elderly and the young – meant that, while it made them somewhat more acceptable to the Labour Party, their yield would be correspondingly low: in the outcome, 60 per cent of all prescriptions were free. Again, Crossman – like Bevan before him, and like his Conservative successor, Sir Keith Joseph – asked his officials to calculate the likely income from a boarding charge to hospital patients, but decided that the administrative and political hassle would outweigh the financial gains. Instead, he argued for greater reliance on the NHS element in the national insurance contributions.

Three aspects of this debate should be noted. First, the debate about the problems of NHS finance did not split neatly into party patterns: Labour and Conservative Ministers were agreed about the nature of the dilemma, although there was some disagreement about possible solutions. Second, debate did not lead to action. In 1964 the incoming Labour Government halved the income from charges: it fell from 5.4 per cent of the total NHS budget in 1963–64 to 2.3 per cent in 1967–68, to rise to 3.5 per cent by the end of the Labour administration's term of office. And it remained at virtually that fig-ure throughout the Conservative administration, from 1970 to 1974. The Labour Government was prevented by economic constraints from carrying out its manifesto pledge of abolishing charges; and the Conservative Government was inhibited by problems of admin-istration from following through its bias towards introducing more

The politics of technocratic change

charges. Both parties were, moreover, too committed to the principle of the NHS to consider any root and branch reforms: not only conflict but policy options were constrained by consensus. Lastly, the growing acceptance by Ministers that demands would always, and inevitably, outrun resources made explicit their rationing role: the fact that central government would inescapably have to make choices between competing priorities. Once again, it is important to stress that this was not a new discovery. But in the 1960s and 1970s, the issue acquired a new salience, helping to shape the way in which specific policy problems were perceived. It is to some of these specific policy problems that we now turn.

PLANNING AND RATIONING

In 1962 the Minister of Health, Enoch Powell, published a Hospital Plan for England and Wales.[29] It was the first attempt since the creation of the NHS to take a 'comprehensive view of the hospital service': to devise a national plan designed to bring about a distribution of hospital beds based not on the haphazard inherited pattern but on centrally-determined criteria for matching resources to needs. Over the next decade, the Hospital Plan envisaged, work would start on building 90 new hospitals and substantially remodelling 134 existing hospitals. The total costs would be, the Plan estimated, £500 million: over three times as much as had been spent in the previous decade and a half. National norms for the appropriate number of beds for each locality were laid down: 3.3 acute beds per 1,000 population. A national pattern of hospitals would be created: District General Hospitals of 600 to 800 beds, each serving a population of 100,000 to 150,000 people. All the required medical expertise would be concentrated in these hospitals; in turn, many existing hospitals would be closed.

The production of the Hospital Plan can usefully be seen as the outcome of two trends. First, exogenous to the NHS, there were the changes in the political environment and administrative styles discussed earlier in this chapter. Second, endogenous to the NHS, there was the gradual creation of a consensus among professionals and others about the need to create a new hospital system. In 1956, as we have seen, the Guillebaud Committee drew attention to the inadequacy of the building programme. In 1959 a group of BMA consultants published a report advocating a ten year hospital plan. A series of research studies and conferences was devoted to the subject of how many beds were needed, and just which specialties

73

should be concentrated in the new District General Hospitals.

The Hospital Plan was thus the child of a marriage between professional aspirations and the new faith in planning: between what might be called medical expertise and administrative technology. It was designed to promote both efficiency and equity: to bring about uniform standards throughout the NHS. But, it is important to stress, the detailed recommendations of the Plan – the basic vision of what a hospital service should be like – were almost entirely determined by the medical consensus: to caricature only slightly, the vision was designed to maximise the quality of medical care being delivered. Within the Ministry the issue of determining norms and the pattern of hospitals was defined largely as a matter for the medical experts: 'a purely scientific thing, where you accept the advice of your medicos', as one of the administrators put it. There is no indication in the Hospital Plan of other possible criteria being considered, such as accessibility for patients or the effect of hospital size on staff morale or recruitment. The domination of the professional definition of the problem being tackled was all the greater for being implicit and unargued.

The point can be further illustrated by a report published in 1969 when a Committee of the Central Health Services Council was asked to examine the functions of the District General Hospital (DGH) in the light of developments since the Hospital Plan.[30] Of the Committee's 18 members, under the lay chairmanship of Sir Desmond Bonham-Carter, 12 were doctors. Their main conclusion was that DGHs should be larger than envisaged in 1962. Again, the dominating criterion was the need to promote technical excellence. No consultant should ever have to work on his own; there should always be teams of two consultants, at the least, in each specialty. Similarly, the 'need for efficient organisation and staffing of supporting technical and other services' pointed in the direction of larger hospitals. So the conclusion drawn was that DGHs should serve populations of between 200,000 and 300,000, so virtually doubling the figure given in the Hospital Plan.

In the event, plans and visions were only partially fulfilled. The capital building programme of the NHS did expand rapidly after 1962: the annual rate of investment more than doubled over the next decade. But it remained vulnerable to the economic crises which punctuated these years: when Chancellors of the Exchequer insisted on cuts in public expenditure, Ministers of Health tended to accept cuts in their capital building programme in return for safeguarding their current budget. Moreover, the recommendations of the Bonham-Carter report were never accepted as official policy. The divergence between plans and achievement marks, in part, also a divergence between administrative and professional definitions of rationality, on the one hand, and political definitions of rationality, on the other. In terms of efficiency, nothing was more destructive than sudden changes in the capital investment programme: precisely the kind of 'chopping and changing' which the Plowden Committee had sought to prevent. Politically, however, cutting the capital programme was far more rational than cutting the current budget: the former meant exporting the loss of jobs into the private sector, while the latter would have meant a confrontation with the constituency of health service providers.

Similarly, politicians were more sensitive to the social costs of building large technological palaces. The argument was sharply put by Crossman[31]:

The great case for the big hospital is first, that the expertise is gathered in one place so that all the specialists who could possibly be interested can be around the bed; and secondly, that size is now necessary for a rational use of expensive equipment. Perfectly true, perfectly true! Of course from the consultants' point of view these huge hospitals are right. But I ask myself about the social cost . . . Nurses were often available for the small local hospital. But if you build a large hospital in the wrong place you won't draw the ladies from the six local small hospitals because they went there part-time from their villages . . . There are all kinds of practical problems of social organisation which seem to me to have been strangely neglected in the planning of the hospital programme.

Moreover, it was Ministers who carried the political costs of closing smaller hospitals made redundant by the development of the new DGHs. For it was Ministers who had to face the constituency protests from communities faced with the loss of their local hospitals.

The implementation of the hospital building programme presents a further puzzle. Why, twenty years after the publication of the Hospital Plan, is its vision of a country studded with modern hospitals still unfulfilled? Why did hospital building enjoy such low priority? For the politician, it might be assumed, there could be no better advertisement than a shining new hospital: a visible symbol of his or her commitment to improving the people's health. For the doctors, as already argued, new hospitals meant the opportunity to practice what the profession considered to be higher quality medicine. For the consumer, in turn, new hospitals surely meant better services with higher standards of treatment. It was Bevan who once remarked that he would rather survive in the stark impersonality of a new hospital than die in the cosy comfort of a cottage hospital. So here there would appear to be a congruence of interests which yet, in the event, was frustrated.

To explore the reasons for this seemingly perverse outcome is to illuminate also some of the special characteristics of the health care policy arena. Let us start with the politicians. If the arena of health care policy was depoliticised to a remarkable degree, one reason for this was that it offered remarkably little scope for the politician seen as a vote maximiser: *homo economicus* in the political market. Negative action, such as stopping the closure of a local hospital, might bring immediate political dividends. Positive action, except when it involved awarding higher pay to NHS employees, could rarely bring such political gains. From time to time, Ministers might announce special action to bring down waiting lists. But, throughout the history of the NHS, the number of people on the waiting lists hovered stubbornly around the 600,000 mark: improving the available services simply encouraged general practitioners to put more patients in the queue. The captain shouted his orders: the crew went on as before. Moreover, there was an inevitable time-lag between Ministerial intervention and outcomes: in effect, Ministers were working for the benefit of their successors. In the case of hospital building, there might be a delay of ten years between sanctioning construction and completion. If we use a vote-maximising model to explain the behaviour of politicians, it is therefore not surprising that the NHS building programme should have received low priority.[32] However, to make this point may also suggest the limitations of such a model: to explain ministerial action – as distinct from ministerial inaction – we may have to see politicians as paternalistic rationalisers, seeking to maximise not votes but rather a certain vision of what the NHS ought to be.

Next, the medical profession did have a general commitment to, and self-interest in, building new hospitals. However, the organisations representing the medical profession, such as the BMA, had a specific and prior interest in maximising the incomes of their members. Indeed their survival as organisations depended on satisfying their members in this respect,[33] as indeed did that of other organisations – trade union and professional – representing NHS workers. They might well argue for greater public investment in the NHS: this, as we have seen, was precisely the strategy adopted by the BMA in the 1960s and it was further followed by the trade unions in the 1970s. Their immediate demands were for more money for their members. If it came to the choice between current and capital spending, then Cabinet decisions were probably an accurate reflection of the priorities of organised labour in the NHS (however much organised labour, unconstrained by the problems of revenue raising, might protest that there should be no need for such a choice).

Lastly, there were the consumers of health care. If these have so far not been discussed as actors in the health care policy arena, it is because for most of the period being discussed they were the ghosts in the NHS machinery: lacking any institutional representation until the creation of Community Health Councils in 1974 (see the concluding section of this chapter). The Regional Hospital Boards and Hospital Management Committees were agents of the Minister: they lacked all legitimacy as representatives of the local community – though some of their members were chosen after consultation with local interests. Even if they had seen their role in terms of aggregating and giving organised expression to local demands for new hospitals – which they did not – they could not have carried conviction. Indeed the history of the NHS is remarkable for the fact that not a single board or authority ever resigned *en bloc* in protest against inadequate funding – or, for that matter, was sacked by the Minister for incompetence. The RHBs and HMCs might lobby and nag Ministers, and they might well harness the support of their local MPs. But overt political action – in the sense of orchestrating a public campaign – was not part of the rules of the game. The NHS was designed, after all, as an organisation for controlling rather than articulating demands. If indeed there was overwhelming satisfaction with the NHS, this may have reflected the service's success in shaping public expectations rather than in being shaped by them.

The implementation of the Hospital Plan is significant from another perspective as well: that of the central–local relationship. On the face of it, the publication of the Plan might be seen as the assertion of central authority designed to bring about national standards throughout the country. In the event, however, it set the pattern for subsequent attempts in the 1970s to introduce national norms of provision: the two priority documents published in the mid 1970s (see chap. 4). Its neat package of norms was subverted by the two principles, implicit in the debate about their implementation, that have haunted all attempts at national planning aimed at achieving uniformity. The first is what might be called the principle of infinite diversity: no two populations or communities are the same, no two consultants practice the same kind of medicine, and thus national norms inevitably have to be adapted to unique, local circumstances. But since no criteria are available to judge precisely how (or by what measures) local populations or consultants differ, we cannot know what divergences from national norms are acceptable or otherwise. The second is what might be called the principle of infinite indeterminacy: the future cannot be predicted, and we therefore cannot know how changes in the population structure, in the childbearing proclivities of families or in medical technology will affect the need for services. Consequently national norms had to be interpreted and adapted flexibly. Indeed national norms themselves had a disconcerting habit of changing, as more or fewer babies were born, as ideas about the number of beds required for any given population changed, as the emphasis switched from providing hospital care to enhancing community care. Moreover it soon became apparent that the very notion of basing planning on bed norms was highly questionable. Providing beds was not, after all, the objective, only the means: the aim, presumably, was to provide services for patients. The services provided for any given population depended on the *way* in which beds were used – the numbers of medical and other staff, the technical facilities available, clinical decisions about the appropriate lengths of stay and so on – rather than on the *number* of beds available. While in theory nothing could be more concrete than norms based on bed numbers, in practice these turned out to be a somewhat metaphysical concept, as it became apparent that the relationship between means and aims was highly problematic and uncertain.

The two principles not only subverted the Plan, in the sense that what finally emerged was much less tidy than orginally envisaged; they also subverted the formal relationship between the centre and the periphery. In theory, the central department could perfectly properly have instructed its agents – the RHBs and HMCs – to carry out its centrally determined plans. In practice, the command structure became a negotiated order.[34] The Department of Health and Social Security, as its civil servants told a Select Committee which inquired into the hospital building programme in 1969, simply did not know enough: 'It is not easy for us centrally . . .to form a judgment of the precise needs of each regional board.'[35] The department could 'advise', 'persuade' and 'discuss' to use the words of the civil servants giving evidence. It could dispatch the department's medical officers to the regions to discuss issues with the doctors there. But it would not dictate. If this ran counter to the constitutional fiction of Ministerial responsibility and authority, it accurately reflected the balance of knowledge in the NHS: to the extent that knowledge was defined to be experiential, judgemental and professional – too complex to be caught in crude statistics – so, inevitably, power lay at the periphery.

There remained the fact that the NHS was financed out of public money: that the Minister was accountable to Parliament for every penny spent. Hence the curious phenomenon, already noted in the 1950s, of a central government department which was often very latitudinarian on major policy issues but which behaved with nit-picking pedantry in matters of detail. If health authorities were permitted considerable freedom to interpret national plans for hospital provision or policy circulars,[36] they were given very much less freedom in interpreting departmental notes about the details of the buildings. If the DHSS could not plan a uniform national service, it is tempting to conclude from the chorus of complaints made by the RHBs to the 1969 Select Committee, it was certainly determined to impose a uniform pattern of cost control. The result was frustration at the periphery: complaints about excessive bureaucracy, about unnecessary delays while plans were repeatedly scrutinised at the centre and about the lack of expertise of a rapidly revolving cast of civil servants.

So the NHS, at the end of the 1960s, presents the spectacle of mutual frustration. The health authorities were frustrated by what they perceived to be excessive interference by central government. Yet central government Ministers felt frustrated by their inability to translate formal power into effective power. To quote Richard Crossman again, reflecting on his experience as Secretary of State at the DHSS:

It was often said to me by Treasury officials when I was Minister, 'Of course we couldn't possibly put the Health Service under local authorities because we wouldn't be able to control the expenditure'. And I always replied, 'But you don't control it today'. Because, of course, you don't have in the Regional Hospital Boards a number of obedient civil servants carrying out the central orders . . . You have a number of powerful, semi-autonomous Boards whose relation to me was much more like the relations of a Persian satrap to a weak Persian Emperor. If the Emperor tried to enforce his authority too far he lost his throne or at least lost his resources or something broke down.[37]

In fact, of course, the Treasury was right: central government did control expenditure. But, similarly, Crossman was right: within the capped budgets allocated to them, the regions enjoyed a large degree of autonomy in the way they allocated their money and organised their services. To a large extent the 1974 reorganisation of the NHS

– the subject of the last section of this chapter – can be seen as an attempt to devise a solution to the problem of mutual frustration.

The sense of frustrated bafflement felt by Ministers can be illustrated by the case of services for the mentally ill. From the start, everyone had agreed that these represented the slum of the NHS: as we saw in the previous chapter, Bevan in 1950 had warned his Cabinet colleagues about the likelihood of scandal breaking about poor conditions in mental hospitals. Almost every politician who succeeded Bevan as Minister of Health proclaimed the need to give priority to improving these services. Yet progress was painfully slow. There was indeed some progress: between 1948 and 1959, spending on psychiatric hospitals accounted for over a quarter of the total capital budget.[38] Yet achievement always lagged behind the targets set by central policy-makers: at the end of the 1960s the objectives set in the Hospital Plan and other public documents had not been met. [39] Much the same was true of other hospitals for the chronically ill, such as for the mentally handicapped. It was not surprising therefore that Crossman in 1969 seized the opportunity provided by a report revealing 'scandalous conditions' at one of these hospitals, Ely.[40] He insisted on publishing an uncensored version. He pressed the RHBs to divert funds into the chronic care sector. He exploited the chance to set up the Hospital Advisory Service (HAS): what was in all but name an inspectorate, reporting directly to the Secretary of State.[41]

The case of the services for the mentally ill, and other chronic care groups, demonstrates the limited ability of the centre to shape the pattern of services at the periphery. Equally important, it once more underlines the extent to which any organisation such as the NHS represents a pressure group for maintaining the inherited pattern. In terms of the medical profession's ladder of prestige, the specialties in the long-stay sector were at the bottom of the hierarchy – whether measured by the number of merit awards handed out or by the proportion of immigrant doctors working in them.[42] Moreover, weakness was self-reinforcing: given their lack of prestige, those working in these services were in no position to assert their claims to more resources effectively. Similarly, the consumers of these services were – by definition – those least able to articulate their demands. In contrast, the users of acute services were well placed to articulate their demands. There is thus no need to invoke a conspiracy theory of medical power to explain the strength of the constituency for the *status quo* in terms of the balance between the acute and the chronic sectors of the NHS. It was Crossman's Conservative successor, Sir Keith Joseph, who identified the alliance of indifference between the medical profession and the lay managers of the NHS. 'There has been no systematic demand for better standards either by the medical or lay elements', he pointed out.[43] Further, he argued, 'Doctors can be remarkably selective in choosing the ills they regard worthy of treatment . . . No one can see better than doctors the needs of the public and the shortcomings of the service. I am not aware that there has been steady, powerful, informed medical pressure to remedy the real worst shortcomings.'

The challenge for Ministers who sought a change in this balance was therefore precisely how to create a political coalition for change: how to give more visibility to the problems of the chronic care sector and to enhance their political salience. Hence Crossman's decision to exploit scandal, despite the reluctance of some of his civil servants who were afraid of the effects on morale in the service. Hence, too, the decision to subsidise MIND (the National Association for Mental Health) – the pressure group concerned with improving conditions in mental health hospitals. This decision may seem perverse: why should Ministers use public money to finance an organisation whose aim was to embarrass them by pointing out shortcomings in the NHS? But the encouragement of this Quangig – quasi-non-governmental-interest-group – makes perfect sense once it is recognised that Ministers needed allies.

Given these problems, it is not surprising to find a move from planning towards rationing by the beginning of the 1970s: precisely the same trend evident in the case of planning for consultant manpower (see previous chapter). The norms of the Hospital Plan and other subsequent documents implied that there was a desirable package of provision for any given population. Further, it assumed that progress towards achieving equity in the geographical distribution of resources could best be achieved through a building programme. Both assumptions became increasingly frayed by experience. Given the principles of infinite diversity and infinite indeterminacy, were norms such a good idea? Given the stuttering progress of the capital building programme, could this be relied on as the instrument for bringing about equity?

Planning by norms was not abandoned until the 1980s (see Ch. 4); but it became diluted. The strategy chosen was to seek a formula for sharing out fairly the available revenue resources: essentially a rationing strategy in that, unlike the planning approach, it did not make any assumptions about the desirable *level* of provision but only about the equitable *share* of the resources to be made available to any given resources. The first such attempt was made in 1970, when a new formula for allocating resources to the regions was introduced.[44] The aim of this was to achieve not equality but equity: allocations weighted by the needs of the population. Subsequently, in 1976, the distributional methodology was further refined: the formula produced by the Resource Allocation Working Party (RAWP) weighed the population primarily by age and mortality factors. Politically, the significance of this approach lay in that it gave public visibility to the existing distribution of resources: inequities which were even more glaring at the sub-regional level.[45] Some regions, notably the London ones, were clearly identified as being (relatively) over-provided. Other regions, such as Trent, were clearly identified as being (relatively) deprived. The development of new analytic methodologies thus gave new salience to the issue of distribution within the NHS: conceptually they solved the puzzle about which criteria should be used to decide who got what, but politically they intensified it.

For the future, the emphasis on greater rationality and equity in the distribution bequeathed two problems: to be discussed in subsequent chapters. First, the formulas might bring about equity in the distribution of resources. But would they bring about equity in access? Would similar bundles of resources in different areas actually mean that the populations served would get the same kind of service and have the same opportunities for treatment? Second, the formulas assumed that progress towards achieving equity could be made painlessly by a process of differential growth: the relatively under-provided regions would simply have a more rapid annual increment of growth than the relatively over-provided regions. No one would suffer. 'I can only equalise on an expanding budget', Crossman had concluded.[46] The commitment to achieving equity thus reflected optimism about the possibilities of economic growth. As that optimism ebbed away during the second half of the 1970s, so the political costs of implementing the new distributional policies increased.

NATIONAL POLICY AND MEDICAL DECISIONS

Implicit in the structure of the NHS was a bargain between the State and the medical profession. While central government controlled the budget, doctors controlled what happened within that budget. Financial power was concentrated at the centre; clinical power was concentrated at the periphery. Politicians in Cabinet made the decisions about how much to spend; doctors made the decisions about which patient should get what kind of treatment. But this implicit bargain represented not so much a final settlement as a truce: an accommodation to what was, for both parties, a necessary rather than a desirable compromise. For central government, there was the dilemma posed by the fact that it carried ultimate responsibility for everything that happened in the NHS. If patients were not treated, Ministers were likely to get the constituency brickbats. But Ministers were in no position to do anything about what might well be the cause of overstretched services: decisions by consultants to keep patients in hospital longer than necessary.[47] All such decisions, although they had crucial implications for the use of NHS resources, belonged to the sacred realm of clinical autonomy. Similarly, the use of ineffective, inefficient or expensive methods of clinical intervention[48] had implications for the NHS as a whole: funds so spent represented opportunities foregone for improving other parts of the NHS – such as the services for the mentally ill and the chronically sick, discussed in the previous section.

The bargain was also frustrating for the medical profession. The price of preserving clinical autonomy – the right of individual doctors to do what they thought right for individual patients – was accepting the constraint of working within fixed budgetary limits. The resources of which doctors disposed were thus limited in a period when the scope for medical intervention was ever-expanding. They might have to work in out-of-date buildings. They might well not get the latest equipment. The medical imperative of maximising the input of care for the individual patient was thus at odds with the financial structure of the NHS. From the 1960s onwards, these ever-present tensions became ever more apparent. To the extent that central government became committed to promoting efficiency and rational planning, so the inhibitions imposed by clinical autonomy became more evident. To the extent that the medical professions's standards were international, so the contrast between what was affordable in a relatively poor country like Britain and in wealthier nations like the United States became more glaring: to a large degree, the frustrations of the medical profession in the 1960s, and even more in the 1970s, were accentuated by the growing gap in national incomes between Britain and its competitors among the advanced industrial nations of the West. Not only was the NHS's share of the national income lower than that of health services in these countries but, perhaps more important, Britain's national income per head was itself falling in relation to that of its competitors.[49] If the medical brain-drain was never large enough to pose a threat to the NHS – which attracted far more doctors from the poorer nations of the Indian sub-continent than it lost to the wealthier societies of North America – it symbolised the shifting economic balance.

The way in which central policy-makers reacted to this situation is significant as much for what they did not do as for what they actually did. Certain policy options were automatically ruled out by the nature of the consensus about the NHS. Thus there was no move towards controlling or even investigating the decisions of clinicians in contrast to the United States, where an open-ended budgetary system led to a series of attempts to introduce a formalised system for reviewing clinical decisions. The doctrine of clinical autonomy continued to reign supreme; significantly, the Health Service Commissioner – whose office was set up in 1974 to deal with patient complaints – was explicitly barred from dealing with cases revolving round questions of clinical judgement. Instead, the preferred strategy was that of persuasion, education and exhortation. At a conference held to celebrate the twentieth anniversary of the foundation of the NHS, Dr Henry Yellowless – Deputy Chief Medical Officer of the Ministry of Health – pointed out that over £2 million a year could be saved if only lengths of stay for patients with appendicitis could be reduced to the same level as that already prevailing in the US: the first of many such exhortations by ministers, civil servants and academics. But, he stressed, 'There can be no question of telling surgeons how long their patients should be in hospital'.[50] All that could be done was to put the surgeons 'in possession of the facts'.

So, consistent with the overall philosophy that developed in the 1960s, there was increasing emphasis on producing better information and on organisational solutions: given better data, given better organisation, more rational decisions would follow – or so it was assumed. A new information system was developed: Hospital Activity Analysis which provided consultants with better information about what they were doing. A new system of medical decision-making within individual hospitals was devised: the so-called Cogwheel system. If all the consultants became aware of the effects of their individual decisions on the total use of resources, it was argued, they would themselves have an incentive to apply pressure on colleagues who used their beds wastefully: it would make it clear that one consultant's extravagance was another consultant's loss. Consultants would view beds no longer as their private property but as a common resource. It is not clear how successful this strategy was. Certainly lengths of stay fell throughout the period in question. But the chorus of exhortations to greater efficiency continued throughout the period in question, as did great variations in practice. The new information system seems to have impinged only marginally on clinical practice; the Cogwheel machinery worked somewhat creakingly.[51] More important, for the purposes of our analysis, is the fact that no other strategy was ever defined to be within the realm of the feasible.

The full complexity and subtlety of the relationship between central policy-makers and clinical decision-makers at the periphery remains to be explored, however. For the paradox is that the centre's lack of authority over clinical decisions could, in some circumstances at least, confer positive advantages on policy-makers: by absolving them from involvement in difficult decisions and by permitting them to shuffle off responsibility for providing extra resources. Two examples illustrate this point: the experience of renal dialysis and of abortion. The case of renal dialysis illustrates the way in which central government could actually control the introduction of a new technology without ever appearing to be infringing medical autonomy. Renal dialysis is an example of a technology which is both expensive and which extends lives: in short, precisely the kind of medical advance which might be expected to generate large demands for extra resources. So, when it became apparent in the early 1960s that this new technology would soon be available, the medical hierarchy of the Ministry of Health took the initiative. A series of conferences – prestigiously chaired by the President of the Royal College of Physicians, Lord Rosenheim – was called. The process of engineering a professional consensus was under way. In the outcome, medical agreement was obtained for what was in all but name a strategy of rationing scarce resources: a policy of concentrating renal dialysis facilities in a limited number of centres – a policy justified, however, not by resource constraints but by medical considerations about the desirability of concentrating expertise. Special resources were set aside for the creation of these centres, but the commitment was limited. The result was, and continues to be, that access to renal dialysis treatment in Britain is limited. Stringent criteria of suitability for treatment are applied: criteria which are more severe than in other countries. Thus in 1975 the number of patients being treated by dialysis (or with a functioning transplant) was 62.0 per 1,000,000 population in Britain, as against 136.1 in Switzerland, 132.4 in Denmark, 102.2 in France, 87.7 in Germany and 85.4 in Sweden.[52] In other words, people in Britain are being turned away to die who, if they lived somewhere else, would be successfully treated. The remarkable fact that the NHS can get away with this politically – that a refusal to save lives does not raise a storm of political protest – demonstrates the positive advantages that central policy-makers can derive from the doctrine of clinical autonomy. For, of course, it is not Ministers or civil servants who decide who should be treated. It is the clinicians concerned. The definition of certain areas of decision-making as being medical – and the consequent diffusion of responsibility for the consequences – thus prevents overload at the centre. The fact that no patient under the NHS system has a legal *right* to any specific kind of treatment – that it is the clinician who determines what the patient 'needs' – means that it is possible to fragment and dissolve national policy issues into a series of local clinical decisions. Political problems are, in effect, converted into clinical problems.

The case of abortion is somewhat different, but raises some of the same issues. The starting point here is the passage of the 1967 Abortion Act: a private member's bill sympathetically encouraged by Ministers. The result was to liberalise the law and to increase the demand for what were now legal operations. However, the Act imposed no responsibility on the Ministry of Health to provide the necessary facilities, nor did it impose on individual consultants a duty to carry out the procedure. To have provided the necessary facilities would have meant finding extra resources. To have imposed a duty on consultants would have infringed the principle of clinical autonomy. The Ministry in fact did neither. As the Lane Committee pointed out in 1974, the central department gave no 'guidance to hospital authorities as to what they consider the reasonable requirement to be in the field of abortion'.[53] The result was wide variation in the facilities provided in 1973 the Newcastle region provided abortions for nearly 90 per cent of the women living in the region who wanted them, while Birmingham recorded a figure of under 20 per cent. If the principle of clinical autonomy gave the central department a pretext for doing nothing, it was the existence of a private market which made this policy of inaction politically feasible. Demand created its own supply: in the private sector. In 1968, 35 per cent of all abortions were carried out by private clinics – some operated for profit, some run by charitable organisations. In 1971 the figure was 43.4 per cent. Central government had found yet another way of absolving itself from the necessity to command or to instruct, as well as from the need to find extra resources.

If it was thus impossible or undesirable to command, might it not have been possible to change the structure of incentives within which doctors worked? A partial answer to this question is provided by the new pay deal negotiated with the general practitioners in 1966: the so-called Family Doctor Charter.[54] The negotiations and the settlement provide an instructive case history, which illuminates both the internal political dynamics of the medical profession and the scope of the Ministry of Health for introducing change.

In 1963 the annual meeting of BMA representatives passed a motion which called for urgent action to 'upgrade the financial status of family doctors'. Implicit in this motion was not just the customary demand for more money but a demand for a change in the structure of medical earnings: the aim was to reduce the differential between general practitioners and consultants. The resentment of general practitioners at being the poor relations of the medical profession within the NHS – of being virtually excluded from the prestigious hospital world of high technology – had broken into the open. The logic of the relationship between general practitioners and consultants was essentially a commercial one: it had been forged in the nineteenth century as a way of regulating the competition between general practitioners and hospital specialists. The referral system then evolved was essentially a demarcation agreement between two crafts, of exactly the same kind that developed between different crafts in shipbuilding and other British industries. General practitioners were the gatekeepers to the whole health care system: all referrals to hospital had to come through them, and they were thus assured of patients. Similarly, once patients were past the gate, consultants took over. Both were thus assured of clients. But while the NHS removed the commercial logic behind this system, it also perpetuated it: hence the frustration of the general practitioners in the 1960s.

The militancy of the general practitioners was embarrassing for the BMA. For it exposed the fact that general practitioners and consultants did not necessarily have the same interests. Yet if the BMA was reluctant to go into battle, others were not. The Medical Practitioners' Union, a body with a long history but a small membership, took up the cause of the general practitioners. A new breakaway General Practitioners' Association was formed. Competition between the various medical organisations fanned militancy. In 1965 the proposals of the impartial review body – set up as a result of the recommendations of the Royal Commission on Doctors' and Dentists' Remuneration (discussed in the previous chapter) – were rejected. In March 1965 the BMA threatened mass resignations by general practitioners from the NHS. At the same time, the BMA published its demands in the form of a 'Charter for the Family Doctor Service'.

The details of the Charter are of no concern here, but some of the main elements should be noted. First, the general practitioners demanded an end to the 'pool' system: that is, spending on general practitioner services should be determined by the number of patients, not by a capped budget. Second, they demanded a new form of contract which would limit their responsibility for their patients to a specified working day and a five and a half day working week: the concept of professional responsibilities for patients being unlimited was to be dropped. Third, they demanded the creation of an independent corporation to provide loans for improving practice premises and equipment. Lastly, they demanded that general practitioners who did not wish to be paid on the basis of capitation fees should have a choice between salaries and item of service fees: that is, payment by the act.

Months of negotiations followed between the profession and the Ministry, headed by Kenneth Robinson. Interestingly the civil servant most immediately involved was Robert Armstrong, a future Cabinet Secretary – evidence perhaps of the infusion of some high-flyers into the Ministry's hierarchy. The compromise that finally emerged in 1966 was a monument to the enduring strength of the underlying consensus about the NHS. The demands of the BMA which would have undermined the basic philosophy of the NHS were effectively ignored. Nothing more was heard of item of service fees, although specific payments were to be paid for some general practitioner work such as night-visiting, vaccinations and immunisations. Similarly, nothing more was heard about limiting the general practitioner's total responsibility for his or her patients. But the pool was abolished. A financial corporation for encouraging investment in general practice was set up, and various modifications in the system of calculating earnings were agreed. In particular, a basic allowance – or salary element – was introduced, as were new incentives for doctors to practice in under-provided areas of the country.

The cost of the settlement to the Ministry of Health was a £24 million a year addition to the cost of general practitioner services. But, in return, the Ministry was able to give new impetus to some long-standing aims of policy. The financial provisions of the settlement were largely designed to promote better quality practice, in terms of improved surgeries, more support staff and encouragement for the formation of group practices: the 1966 settlement marks the beginning of a boom in Health Centres.[55] These, as noted in Chapter

1, had been the centre piece of planning for general practice before the creation of the NHS. Subsequently, a combination of medical hostility and financial stringency had consigned them to a policy limbo. A combination of changes in medical attitudes and the easing of budgetary constraints had created new opportunities for central policy-makers to push a policy consistent not only with the ideological bias of the Labour Ministry of Health, but also with the efficiency bias of the technocratic rationalisers. The Family Doctor Charter negotiations thus provide a case study both of the limits on the potential for change, imposed by the prevailing consensus, and the opportunities to influence clinical practice through the use of incentives.

The history of these negotiations also underlines a trend which was to emerge increasingly strongly over the next decade: the ever-deepening divisions within the medical profession. In the 1960s, in contrast to the 1950s and again the 1970s, doctors did well for themselves financially. In 1972 the Review Body reported that 'the medical profession, taken as a whole, gained ground rather than lost it in relation to other workers' between the publication of the Royal Commission report and 1971.[56] There were, inevitably, battles between the profession and the Government, particularly when the recommendations of the Review Body ran counter to incomes policy: indeed in 1970 the Review Body resigned because of the Government's refusal to implement its recommendations fully. Pay, inevitably, could not be de-politicised in the NHS. Equally important, however, were the battles within the medical profession. In 1966 the Junior Hospital Doctors' Association was formed, successfully beginning a campaign to raise salaries which was to end by threatening the differentials between consultants and their supporting cast of doctors. Increasingly, too, the Hospital Consultants' and Specialists' Association – founded in 1948 but largely dormant until the end of the 1960s – began to challenge the right of the BMA to act as the voice of the consultants: in 1974 it unsuccessfully applied to the Industrial Relations Court for negotiating rights.[57]

These fissions helped to expose the weaknesses in the machinery of professional corporatism within the NHS. On paper, the structure was highly corporate, with the medical profession being organised in clearly defined associations and with a highly centralised negotiating structure. In practice, the associations found it difficult to deliver the goods: indeed by 1972, the BMA had become sufficiently anxious to invite a former chairman of ICI, Sir Paul Chambers, to investigate its constitution and organisation.[58] Under the veneer of

disciplined corporatism, however, the reality was an anarchic syndicalism. The leaders of the medical profession – the bureaucrats of
the BMA and others – faced precisely the same nagging difficulty
as the paternalistic rationalisers at the Ministry of Health: how to
influence, let alone control, the individualistic practitioners at the
periphery. If the relationship between the professional élite and the
bureaucratic élite was an intimate one,[59] it was at least in part
because they shared the same problem: that of corporatist rationalisers trying to cope with a syndicalist constituency.

IN SEARCH OF AN ORGANISATIONAL FIX

The original structure of the NHS, everyone agreed, had one fundamental, inbuilt weakness. This was the administrative separation
of the hospital, general practitioner and local authority health services: a structure which reflected political expediency, not administrative logic. It is therefore not surprising that the issue of
organisational reform surged back onto the political agenda in the
1960s, and that finally in 1974 a reorganised NHS emerged. Not
only were these the years of faith in the ability of organisational
change to promote greater efficiency and effectiveness in all spheres
of government. As already noted, there was also increasing frustration within the NHS at the seeming inability of central government
to implement its policies. If there was to be rational planning, then
an appropriate administrative machinery had to be designed. If a
further spur to action was needed, then there was the growing
emphasis on co-ordinating hospital and community services in order
to minimise the costs of caring for an ageing population. Once again,
change was anchored in consensus. By 1968 when Kenneth Robinson, the Labour Minister of Health, published the first consultative
document on reorganisation, the need for administrative reform had
become part of the conventional wisdom. The agreement spanned
the political parties, and reflected also the views of the medical
profession: already in 1962 the report of the Porritt Committee, set
up by the medical profession, had come out in favour of a unified
health service based on area boards. Once again, however, consensus
both made change possible and constrained its scope. For it embodied notions not only about what was desirable but also about the
limits of political feasibility.

In principle, the Labour and Conservative parties were agreed
that a unified health and local authority system would be the ideal
solution: all the more so, since there was a great deal of comple-

mentarity and substitution between the health and welfare services, particularly for the elderly. Further, they were agreed that the best way of achieving this ideal would be to transfer the health services to local government. However, both parties were at one in accepting that such a solution was not feasible: that there was no point in even putting it on the agenda of possible policy options. In part, this was a tribute to the veto-power of the medical profession, with its tradition of entrenched hostility to local government control. While this issue was central to the medical profession, it was peripheral to the local government lobby: although local authorities were naturally in favour of taking over health services, their diffuse support would not outweigh the concentrated opposition that could be expected from the doctors. In part, too, the rejection of the local government option marked a recognition of the practical problems involved. Such a transfer of power would have required basic changes in both the money-raising capacities of local government and in its boundaries. However, it is also worth noting that another option was also ruled out of court: that of transferring local government welfare services to the NHS – an option suggested by the logic of complementarity and substitutability. If the medical profession had veto power, so did the local government lobby. The search for an organisational solution to the NHS's problems can therefore be best understood as policy-making under constraints, where the ideal was often seen as the enemy of the feasible: the politics of the second-best.[60]

There were two further ingredients in the consensus. First, there was agreement that, since it was not possible to amalgamate health and local government services, the best available solution would be to align the boundaries of health and local authorities: the assumption being that co-habitation would lead to co-ordination. Second, there was agreement that the aim of reorganisation should be to promote better management: to give more power, as it were, to the paternalistic rationalisers, and to create more scope for the rational analysis and efficient solution of problems.

Given these shared assumptions, it is hardly surprising that the successive proposals put forward – from Kenneth Robinson's 1968 consultative document to Sir Keith Joseph's 1974 final solution – show a remarkable degree of continuity, only marginally affected by party ideology. The proposals did change in detail, but the changes were prompted as much by developments in the external environment of the NHS as by party considerations. The 'central theme' of the 1968 Green Paper was unification.[61] The new NHS was to be based on 40 to 50 Area Boards, responsible for all health services, including the general practitioner services: a number chosen because it was expected that the Royal Commission on Local Government would recommend the creation of 40 to 50 local authorites. All other NHS authorities – including the regions – would disappear. The style of the Area Boards would be managerial. Their membership would be small; and while 'some members with broad professional knowledge of medical and related services would be needed', the representation of 'special interests' was specifically excluded. The senior officers of the Board would act as an executive directorate, with the Chief Administrator acting as Managing Director.

In 1970 Richard Crossman, now in charge of NHS reorganisation as Secretary of State of the DHSS, published yet another Green Paper.[62] The most obvious change from the 1968 document was prompted by events outside the control of the NHS: the decision to base the new system of local government not on 40 to 50 authorities but on about 90. So, given the agreement on the need for co-terminosity, this implied 90 Area Health Authorities. In turn, this raised the question of whether one central department could effectively control this number of authorities. Crossman was anxious to knock out the regional tier altogether[63]; his civil servants were less enthusiastic. In the event the Green Paper fudged the issue: it envisaged the creation of 14 Regional Health Councils with somewhat vague co-ordinating and planning roles. Crucially, however, these Councils were not to be a link in the administrative chain of command: the DHSS would deal directly with the Areas: 'The central Department will need to concern itself more closely than in the past with the expenditure and efficiency of the administration at the local level.'

The 1970 Green Paper was significant also for its attempts to meet some of the criticisms prompted by its predecessor, and its concessions to various interest groups. The managerial emphasis of the 1968 Green Paper had antagonised the medical profession, among others. For example, the *British Medical Journal* commented that 'A case for such a drastic curtailment of the participation of the public and of the profession in the management of the NHS might be made simply in the interests of efficiency. But there is a limit to the extent to which the principles of organisation and methods should be introduced into a medical service'[64], a curious echo of Morrison's protest, in the 1946 Cabinet debates, about using the efficiency argument as the determining criterion in health services organisation. Nor had local government been pleased. In response, Crossman introduced the principle of representative membership for the new health authorities: one-third of the members were to be appointed by the health profession, one-third appointed by the local authorities and one-third plus the chairman appointed by the Secretary of State. This proposal was pushed through only after a bitter battle with the Treasury, which argued that the appointment of members by interest groups was incompatible with the accountability of health authorities to Parliament. Finally, the 1970 Green Paper argued that 'there must be more, not less, local participation' in the reorganised NHS, and to this end proposed the creation of district committees 'on which people drawn from the local community and people working in the local health service can contribute to the work of running the district's services' (in ways unspecified).

The Labour Government, and Crossman with it, were voted out of office before these proposals could be implemented. In 1971 Crossman's Conservative successor at the DHSS, Sir Keith Joseph, published his Consultative Document, followed by a White Paper in 1972, legislation in 1973 and the unveiling of the new NHS in 1974. Two linked themes shaped Sir Keith's approach. First, as the Consultative Document put it, there was the emphasis on 'effective management'[65] – harking back to the 1968 Green Paper. Second, there was the need to correct the 'imbalances and gaps', to quote the 1972 White Paper[66], in the provision of NHS services: to redress the balance between the acute and the chronic services in favour of the latter. Effective management would be the tool used to achieve this objective. Hitherto, the White Paper argued, 'There has been no identified authority whose task it has been . . .to balance needs and priorities rationally and to plan and provide the right combination of services for the benefit of the public.' In future, the new Area Health Authorities (AHAs) would perform this role. They would identify the 'real needs' of the population, order priorities, work out plans and assess their effectiveness.

The new NHS that emerged in 1974 was different in a number of respects from that envisaged under the Labour Green Paper. First, the Regional authorities re-emerged as executive agencies, the link between the DHSS and the Area Health Authorities in the chain of command: any attempt by the DHSS to control the AHAs directly – the 1972 White Paper argued, reflecting the views of the civil service – would lead to 'over-centralisation and delay'. Second, a new tier was inserted into the hierarchy of administration: larger AHAs were to be divided into districts, each run by a team of officers on a consensus basis (thus giving each member, including representa-

THE CHANGING ADMINISTRATIVE STRUCTURE OF THE NATIONAL HEALTH SERVICE (ENGLAND)

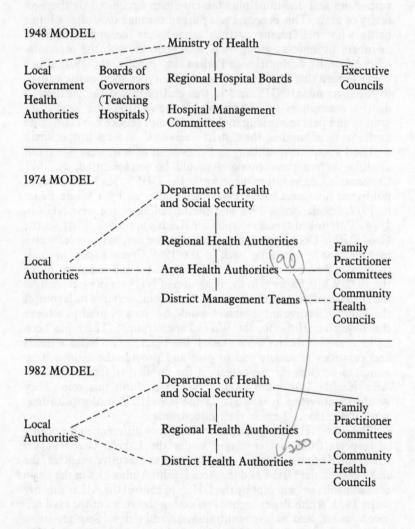

1948 MODEL

Ministry of Health

Local Government Health Authorities	Boards of Governors (Teaching Hospitals)	Regional Hospital Boards	Executive Councils
		Hospital Management Committees	

1974 MODEL

Department of Health and Social Security

Regional Health Authorities

Local Authorities ———— Area Health Authorities *(90)* ———— Family Practitioner Committees

District Management Teams – – – – Community Health Councils

1982 MODEL

Department of Health and Social Security

Local Authorities

Regional Health Authorities ———— Family Practitioner Committees

District Health Authorities *(200)* – – – – Community Health Councils

——— Indicates line of direct managerial authority
– – – – Indicates consultative/co-ordinating relationships

tives of the local consultants and general practitioners, a right of veto over decisions). This innovation was designed to meet the problems caused by the fact that the boundaries of the AHAs were determined by the doctrine of co-terminosity and thus by decisions about the size and pattern of local government, not by decisions based on the administrative logic of the NHS. Thirdly, every tier in the administrative hierarchy – region, AHA and district – was festooned with professional advisory committees, to ensure that decisions would be made 'in the full knowledge of expert opinion': expert opinion being defined as that of doctors, opticians, pharmacists and nurses. Lastly, the reorganised NHS included an institutional innovation: Community Health Councils (CHCs), one for each of the 200 districts. There was thus to be a division of labour: members of AHAs were intended to manage, while members of CHCs were meant to 'represent the views of the consumer'.

The 1974 reorganisation had a number of characteristics which are worth exploring further, not only for the insights they provide into the problems and dilemmas of policy-making but also for their long-term implications. Most self-evidently, it set the 'voice of the expert' into the concrete of the institutional structure even more firmly than Bevan's design had done. Not only did doctors (and nurses, for the first time) have representation on both the regional and area authorities. Not only was an elaborate multi-tiered machinery devised for articulating professional opinion. But, as we have also seen, the basic unit of management – the District Management Team – gave the representatives of the medical profession veto rights. These extensive concessions should be seen not so much as a victory for the corporate organisations of the medical profession as an acknowledgment of the reality of medical syndicalism. Since decisions at the periphery depended on the active co-operation of the doctors concerned, as the people who determined who got what, it seemed only logical to build the participation of the medical profession into the process of the decision-making machinery. Participation followed effective power.

In conceding representation to the medical profession on health authorities, Joseph was of course only following the Labour Green Paper. Similarly, in line with the Crossman proposals, the 1974 NHS provided for representation of local government interests: a third of AHA members were nominated by local authorities. In both respects, Joseph was forced to compromise the underlying principle of his vision: managerial efficiency. His Consultative Document had firmly stated that 'it would be inappropriate for the authorities to

The politics of the National Health Service

be composed on the representational basis proposed in the 1970 Green Paper'. The main criterion for the selection of members was to be 'management ability'. But, to quote one of Joseph's civil servants, it turned out to be difficult to recruit people with business experience. 'Once you had run through his friends, you had no one else . . . In any case you couldn't have 15 hard-faced businessmen running the AHAs'. Moreover, the medical profession and the local government lobby, backed by the Secretary of State of the Environment, were pressing for representation. So the issue was fudged. To the last the Secretary of State stressed that no one served on health authorities in a representative capacity, but the argument seemed increasingly strained as he made concessions on the methods of selection.

Paradoxically it was also the doctrine of managerial efficiency which led to the institutionalisation of the voice of the consumer, in the shape of Community Health Councils.[67] The role of members in the authorities created in 1948 had never been precisely defined: the implicit presumption was that they would combine the managerial role, as the Minister's agents, with that of articulating the interests of consumers and the local community. But what if the two roles conflicted? The report of the Ely inquiry into abuse in a hospital for the mentally handicapped, cited above, had suggested that the members of the Hospital Management Committee responsible had been more concerned to maintain staff morale than to safeguard the interests of the patients. So, given the new emphasis on the exclusively managerial role of the authority members, it seemed only logical to invent a special institution to voice consumer views: an institution which would have no managerial responsibilities. In logic, the distinction was clear; in practice, particularly given the representation of local authorities on AHAs, it often proved blurred.

Community Health Councils were notable for another feature as well. They represented a further attempt to devise a constituency for the deprived client groups in the NHS: precisely those who, as argued above, would be least able to articulate their demands. Half their members were to be appointed by local authorities; a further sixth by the Regional Health Authorities (as the Regional Hospital Boards now became). But a third were to be chosen by local voluntary bodies, with special emphasis on those representing the elderly, the mentally ill and handicapped, and other deprived groups. The constitution of CHCs is thus a good example of the paternalistic rationalisers deliberately loading the dice of representation in order to achieve a greater measure of justice as between the different client groups of the NHS.

The 1974 reorganisation is significant also for what it reveals about the changing balance of political power within the medical profession. In one crucial respect, the 1974 unification of the NHS was a fiction. General practitioner services remained an autonomous enclave. Some of the members of the new Family Practitioner Committees (FPCs), which administered general practitioner services as the successors to the Executive Councils, were indeed appointed by the AHAs. Furthermore, FPCs and AHAs shared the same administrative boundaries. But half their members were nominated by the professions and financially they dealt directly with the DHSS. At the margins, AHAs might be able to exercise some leverage, through their control over the development of Health Centres and of nursing and other staff attached to general practice. Essentially, however, FPCs were independent bodies: the integration of hospital and primary care services remained a distant dream. In short, general practitioners had successfully asserted their right of veto: their power was measured in terms of what was not done, because it was defined to be outside the realm of the politically feasible.

In contrast, the 1974 reorganisation did mark one important step towards integration: the prestigious teaching hospitals lost their special independent status. Boards of Governors disappeared; teaching hospitals were integrated into the administrative structure of the NHS. Ministers were lobbied hard. Tory peers were strongly represented among the chairmen of the Boards of Governors; the Royal Colleges, too, added their voices to the protests. But all to no avail. The contrast between 1948 and 1974 is striking. While Bevan had had to make extensive concessions to the leaders of the specialists (see ch. 1), Joseph was able virtually to ignore the special pleadings of the consultant élite. Not only had that élite been diluted by the expansion of consultant numbers; equally, it had also become more heterogenous, as it became apparent that consultants at London Teaching Hospitals did not necessarily have the same interests as those at provincial district general hospitals. There could be no clearer warning against using simple-minded élite theories to explain the evolution of policy in the NHS.

So, in 1974, the network of NHS authorities set up in 1948 was swept away. In place of 700 different authorities – Regional Hospital Boards, Boards of Governors, Hospital Management Committees and Executive Councils – there was now a streamlined structure.

There were 15 Regional Health Authorities, 90 Area Health Authorities each with its linked Family Practitioner Committee, and 200 District Management Teams each flanked by a Community Health Council. The change prompted two major lines of criticism. First, the new model NHS was attacked as being excessively managerialist: 'I say to the Secretary of State that his managerialism is terrifying', Crossman proclaimed in a House of Commons debate.[68] Second, the new model NHS was criticised for its excessive bureaucratic complexity. There were too many tiers of administrative authority: the DHSS, the regions, the areas and the districts. 'I am appalled by the prospect of a tremendous block of bureaucrats desiccating every original proposal and being difficult over every case', Crossman added.

In a sense the two criticisms are self-cancelling. If the design of the 1974 NHS had been inspired solely by considerations of managerial efficiency, it would not have taken the complex shape it did. Sir Keith Joseph did bring a firm of management consultants, McKinseys, into the DHSS to advise on the details of the reorganisation. But their influence is reflected chiefly in the rhetoric of reorganisation: in the jargon that clothed the proposals and in the small print of the administrative arrangements with their emphasis on functional management – chains of command based on professional expertise.[69] Some of the strongest opposition within the DHSS to the proposed reorganisation came from the business executives, whom the Prime Minister had brought into government precisely in order to promote greater managerial efficiency. From their point of view, the weakness of the NHS derived largely from the hegemony of the civil servants: as one of them put it, 'It was like pre-1914 Russia – a French speaking élite who couldn't speak Russian'. The real need was to allow 'health service people to run the health service at the top', to end the situation 'where everyone was interfering with everyone else at different levels' and to 'delayer' the NHS by chopping off the regions.

In the event, Sir Keith Joseph ignored the advice of these managerialists. If indeed the new model NHS emerged as an extremely complex structure, it was because he was trying to achieve a variety of policy aims, while seeking to preserve consensus and to avoid conflict. The regional tier was perpetuated partly to avoid conflict with the civil servants, and partly because the administrative boundaries of the AHAs did not provide a satisfactory basis for planning health services. In turn, the district level had to be invented because the AHAs were in many cases too large for a health service based on

The politics of technocratic change

the concept of the District General Hospital. Finally, the elaborate cobweb of advisory committees was added in order to keep the professions happy.

Essentially, therefore, the 1974 reorganisation can be seen as a political exercise in trying to satisfy everyone and to reconcile conflicting policy aims: to promote managerial efficiency but also to satisfy the professions, to create an effective hierarchy for transmitting national policy but also to give scope to the managers at the periphery. The intention was summed up in the slogan of 'maximum delegation downward, maximum accountability upward'. The phrase summed up the nature of the policy problem; but it did not provide a solution. And the politics of disillusionment of the second half of the 1970s – the theme of the next chapter – can in part at least be understood as the natural reaction to this attempt to square the circle. As it turned out, the attempt to please everyone satisfied no one.

REFERENCES

1. The source for all quotations from election manifestos is: F. W. S. Craig (ed.), *British General Election Manifestos, 1900–1974*, Macmillan: London 1975.
2. OFFICE OF HEALTH ECONOMICS, *Efficiency in the Hospital Service*, OHE: London 1967.
3. G. R. SEARLE, *The Quest for National Efficiency*, Blackwell: Oxford 1971.
4. HAROLD MACMILLAN, *The Middle Way*, Macmillan: London 1938.
5. For an account of economic policy during this period, see Samuel Brittan, *Steering the Economy*, Secker & Warburg: London 1969.
6. SECRETARY OF STATE FOR ECONOMIC AFFAIRS, *The National Plan*, HMSO: London 1965, Cmnd. 2764.
7. THE PRIME MINISTER AND MINISTER FOR THE CIVIL SERVICE, *The Reorganisation of Central Government*, HMSO: London 1970, Cmnd. 4506.
8. For the origins of the PESC system, see Sir Richard Clarke, *Public Expenditure Management and Control*, Macmillan: London 1978.
9. CHANCELLOR OF THE EXCHEQUER, *Control of Public Expenditure*, HMSO: London 1961, Cmnd. 1432.
10. COMMITTEE ON THE CIVIL SERVICE, *Report*, HMSO: London 1968, Cmnd. 3638.

11. ROYAL COMMISSION ON LOCAL GOVERNMENT IN ENGLAND, *Report*, HMSO: London 1969, Cmnd. 4040.
12. RUDOLF KLEIN, 'The Politics of Public Expenditure', *British Journal of Political Science*, vol. 6, pt. 4, Oct. 1976, pp. 401–32.
13. As in the previous chapter, the source for all time-series data on NHS expenditure is: Royal Commission on the National Health Service, *Report*, HMSO: London 1979, Cmnd. 7615.
14. Stendhal, *De L'Amour*, Editions de Cluny: Paris 1938, p. 43: 'Ce que j'appelle cristallisation, c'est l'opération de l'esprit, qui tire de tout ce qui se présente la découverte que l'object aimé a de nouvelles perfection.' Translating this into the language of policy analysis, we might freely render this as: 'What I call crystallisation is the operation of the mind which draws out of the environment the discovery that there is a problem demanding attention.'
15. J. ENOCH POWELL, *Medicine and Politics*, Pitman Medical: London 1966.
16. THOMAS MCKEOWN, *The Role of Medicine*, Nuffield Provincial Hospitals Trust: London 1976.
17. A. O. HIRSCHMAN, *Exit, Voice and Loyalty*, Harvard U. P.: Cambridge, Mass. 1970. The Hirschman model applies, of course, to consumers of services only. For the argument that, in the circumstances of the NHS, it also applies to producers, see Rudolf Klein, 'Models of Man and Models of Policy', *Health and Society*, vol. 58, no. 3, 1980, pp. 416–29.
18. ROYAL COMMISSION ON THE NATIONAL HEALTH SERVICE, *op. cit.* (see ref. 13)
19. For perhaps the earliest diagnosis of the dilemma, see F. Roberts, *The Cost of Health*, Turnstile Press: London 1952. Quoted in Robert J. Maxwell, *Health and Wealth*, Lexington Books: Lexington, Mass. 1981. Dr Roberts argued that: 'The expense of the health service is incurred by individuals acting singly; the bill is paid by individuals acting collectively. There is therefore a permanent conflict between the demand for greater expenditure and the demand for smaller expenditure.'
20. JAMES M. BUCHANAN, *The Inconsistencies of the National Health Service*, Institute of Economic Affairs: London 1965. See also Arthur Seldon, *After the NHS*, Institute of Economic Affairs: London 1968.
21. See, for example, B. Abel-Smith, *Value for Money in Health Services*, Heinemann: London 1976.
22. RUDOLF KLEIN, 'The Conflict Between Professionals, Con-

sumers and Bureaucrats', *Journal of the Irish Colleges of Physicians and Surgeons*, vol. 6, no. 3, Jan. 1977, pp. 88–91.

23. DAVID OWEN, *In Sickness and In Health*, Quartet: London 1976.
24. HENRY MILLER, 'In Sickness and In Health: A Doctor's View of Medicine in Britain', *Encounter*, April 1967, pp. 10– 21
25. BRITISH MEDICAL ASSOCIATION, *Health Services Financing*, BMA: London 1969. Note that the title page carries the disclaimer: 'The contents of this report do not necessarily reflect BMA policy.'
26. DOUGLAS HOUGHTON, *Paying for the Social Services*, Institute of Economic Affairs: London 1968.
27. RICHARD CROSSMAN, *Paying for the Social Services*, Fabian Society: London 1969.
28. RICHARD CROSSMAN, *The Diaries of a Cabinet Minister*, vol. 2, p. 707, Hamish Hamilton and Jonathan Cape: London 1976.
29. MINISTER OF HEALTH, *A Hospital Plan for England and Wales*, HMSO: London 1962, Cmnd. 1604. The evolution of this plan has been admirably analysed in David E. Allen, *Hospital Planning*, Pitman Medical: Tunbridge Wells 1979, and my discussion of the document draws heavily on this source.
30. DEPARTMENT OF HEALTH AND SOCIAL SECURITY, *The Functions of the District General Hospital*, HMSO: London 1969.
31. RICHARD CROSSMAN, *A Politician's View of Health Service Planning*, University of Glasgow 1972.
32. For an interesting attempt to apply this kind of model to the NHS, see Cotton M. Lindsay, *National Health Issues: The British Experience*, Hoffmann-La Roche Inc: Santa Monica, CA 1980. One of the conclusions drawn in this study is that the distribution of capital expenditure can, in part, be explained by a vote-buying strategy: that is, money went disproportionately to those regions with a high proportion of marginal constituencies. But the unit of analysis, the region, seems too large and heterogeneous to put much weight on this conclusion.
33. For organisational incentives, see M. Olson, *The Logic of Collective Action*, Harvard U. P.: Cambridge, Mass. 1965.
34. I owe this phrase to W. J. M. Mackenzie, *Power and Responsibility in Health Care*, Oxford U. P. 1979.
35. ESTIMATES COMMITTEE, *Hospital Building in Great Britain: Minutes of Evidence*, HMSO: London 1970, H.C. 59.
36. ROSEMARY STEWART and JANET SLEEMAN, *Continuously Under Review*, Bell: London 1967.
37. RICHARD CROSSMAN, *A Politician's View, op. cit.*

The politics of the National Health Service

38. DEPARTMENT OF HEALTH AND SOCIAL SECURITY, *Review of Health Capital*, DHSS: London 1979.
39. ALAN MAYNARD and RACHEL TINGLE, 'The Objectives and Performance of the Mental Health Services in England and Wales in the 1960s', *Journal of Social Policy*, vol. 4, no. 2, April 1975, pp. 155–168.
40. COMMITTEE OF INQUIRY into Allegations of Ill-Treatment of Patients and Other Irregularities at the Ely Hospital, Cardiff, *Report*, HMSO: London 1969, Cmnd. 3975. For Crossman's own account of how he handled the report, and the subsequent setting up of the HAS, see Richard Crossman, *The Dairies of a Cabinet Minister*, vol. 3. pp. 409ff, Hamish Hamilton and Jonathan Cape: London 1977. See also Rudolf Klein, 'Policy Problems and Policy Perceptions in the National Health Service', *Policy and Politics*, vol. 2, no. 3, 1974, pp. 219–36.
41. RUDOLF KLEIN and PHOEBE HALL, *Caring for Quality in the Caring Services*, Centre for Studies in Social Policy: London 1975.
42. For distinction awards, see P. Bruggen and S. Bourne, 'Further Examination of the Distinction Awards System in England and Wales', *British Medical Journal*, 26 Feb. 1976, pp. 536–7. For immigrant doctors, see Royal Commission on the National Health Service, *op. cit.*, Table 14.6. This shows that, for example, overseas born doctors held 40.9 per cent of all consultant posts in geriatric medicine and 23.4 per cent in mental illness, as against 8.0 per cent in general medicine and 8.3 per cent in surgery.
43. SIR KEITH JOSEPH, 'Marsden Lecture', reprinted as 'Sir Keith Surveys the NHS: Achievements and Failures', *British Medical Journal*, 1 Dec. 1973, pp. 561–2.
44. For an analysis of the resources allocation formulas, see Martin Buxton and Rudolf Klein, *Allocating Health Resources*, Royal Commission on the National Health Service, Research Paper no. 3, London: HMSO 1978.
45. MARTIN BUXTON and RUDOLF KLEIN, 'Distribution of Hospital Provision', *British Medical Journal*, 8 Feb. 1975, pp. 345–9. This analysis showed that the distribution of hospital resources by Area Health Authorities in terms of per capita income varied from 74 per cent *below* the national average to 62 per cent *above* the national average.
46. RICHARD CROSSMAN, *A Politician's View, op. cit.*
47. R. F. L. LOGAN, J. S. A. ASHLEY, R. E. KLEIN, and D. M. ROBSON,

Dynamics of Medical Care: The Liverpool Study into Use of Hospital Resources, London School of Hygiene & Tropical Medicine Memoir no. 14: London 1972.

48. A. L. COCHRANE, *Effectiveness and Efficiency*, Nuffield Provincial Hospitals Trust: London 1972.

49. For comparative statistics of health expenditure, see Organisation for Economic Co-operation and Development, *Public Expenditure on Health*, OECD: Paris 1977.

50. DEPARTMENT OF HEALTH AND SOCIAL SECURITY, NHS Twentieth Anniversary Conference, *Report*, HMSO: London 1968.

51. GORDON MCLACHLAN (ed.), *In Low Gear?*, Oxford U. P. 1971.

52. OFFICE OF HEALTH ECONOMICS, *Renal Failure*, OHE: London 1978.

53. COMMITTEE on the working of the Abortion Act, *Report*, HMSO: London 1974, Cmnd. 5579.

54. Excellent accounts of this episode, which have been drawn upon in the text, can be found in: Rosemary Stevens, *Medical Practice in Modern England*, Yale U. P.: New Haven, Conn. 1966, and Gordon Forsyth, *Doctors and State Medicine*, Pitman Medical: London 1973.

55. PHOEBE HALL, HILARY LAND, ROY PARKER and ADRIAN WEBB, *Change, Choice and Conflict in Social Policy*, Heinemann: London 1975. See Ch. 11; 'The Development of Health Centres' by Phoebe Hall.

56. REVIEW BODY ON DOCTORS' AND DENTISTS' REMUNERATION, *Report 1972*, HMSO: London 1972, Cmnd. 5010.

57. KEITH BARNARD and KENNETH LEE, *Conflicts in the National Health Service*, Croom Helm: London 1977. See Ch. 2, 'Medical Autonomy: Challenge and Responses', by Mary Ann Elston.

58. SIR PAUL CHAMBERS, *Report of an Inquiry into the Association's Constitution and Organization*, reprinted in British Medical Journal, vol. 2, 1977, pp. 45–67.

59. Here I follow Eckstein, *Pressure Group Politics, op cit.* For an analysis of the relationship between the two élites, see Barbara Evans, 'Corridors of Power', *World Medicine*, 10 March 1970, pp. 21–33, and Barbara Evans, 'Power Maze or Party Game', *World Medicine*, 28 Jan. 1976, pp. 17–22.

60. RUDOLF KLEIN, 'NHS Reorganisation: The Politics of the Second Best', *The Lancet*, 26 August 1972, pp. 418–20; Rudolf Klein, 'Policy Making in the National Health Service', *Political Studies*, vol. XXII, no. 1, March 1974, pp. 1–14. This account of reorganisation draws on both sources.

61. MINISTRY OF HEALTH, *National Health Service: The Administrative Structure of the Medical and Related Services in England and Wales*, HMSO: London 1968.

62. DEPARTMENT OF HEALTH AND SOCIAL SECURITY, *National Health Service: The Future Structure of the National Health Service*, HMSO: London 1970.

63. RICHARD CROSSMAN, *The Diaries of a Cabinet Minister*, vol. 3, *op. cit.*, p. 753.

64. Cited in Klein, 1974, *op. cit.*

65. DEPARTMENT OF HEALTH AND SOCIAL SECURITY, *National Health Service Reorganisation: Consultative Document*, DHSS: London 1971.

66. SECRETARY OF STATE FOR SOCIAL SERVICES, *National Health Service Reorganisation: England*, HMSO: London 1972, Cmnd. 5055.

67. RUDOLF KLEIN and JANET LEWIS, *The Politics of Consumer Representation*, Centre for Studies in Social Policy: London 1976.

68. HOUSE OF COMMONS HANSARD, *Parliamentary Debates*, vol. 853, no. 86, 27 March 1973.

69. DEPARTMENT OF HEALTH AND SOCIAL SECURITY, *Management Arrangements for the Reorganised National Health Service*, HMSO: London 1972.

Chapter four
THE POLITICS OF DISILLUSIONMENT

If the start of the 1970s saw the apotheosis of paternalistic rationalism, with the 1974 reorganisation of the NHS as its monument, the second half of the decade produced the politics of disillusionment. Designed in an era of faith in problem-solving through expertise, the reorganised NHS began life at a time when technical questions increasingly became redefined as political issues. With apt symbolism, the 1980s were to begin with the demolition squads moving in to begin chipping away at the monument itself: the reorganised NHS was being reorganised yet again. Cocooned in consensus for the first thirty five years of its existence, the arena of health care policy was gradually opening up as internal conflicts grew more pronounced and external pressures became more intense. If internal conflicts had previously been constrained by consensus, now these conflicts were slowly beginning to fray the consensus itself.

Two sets of factors contributed to this transformation. Within the arena of health care policy, there was the intensification of the trends noted in the previous chapter: in particular, the growing numbers, assertiveness and competitiveness of the actors involved. A stage where once the leaders of the medical profession had been able to soliloquise with little interruption had now become crowded with actors all clamouring to be heard. External to the health care arena, there was the dismaying discovery that the post-war years of economic growth were over, as Britain grappled with the twin problems of recession and inflation. In turn, the new economic situation created a new political climate reflected in the increased ideological polarisation of the Labour and Conservative parties. So demands generated from within the health care arena were increasing at precisely the time when the capacity of the governmental system to accommodate them was falling. Conversely, the ability of the health care system to adapt itself to the new economic and political environment was declining as the multiplication of veto power made the implementation of change more difficult: the snaffle was more in evidence than the horse. By the end of the 1970s, the NHS was more than ever a paradigm of British society as a whole: the stalemate society.[1]

Next, therefore, we shall examine in more detail both sides of this equation: the changes in the health care policy arena on the one hand, and those in its economic and political environment on the other. For it is precisely the relationship between the internally generated demands and the externally enforced pressures which provides the key to the politics of disillusionment.

THE POLITICS OF ECONOMIC CRISIS: THE NHS IN A NEW ENVIRONMENT

For most of the post-war period in Britain, economic growth was the solvent of political conflict. Britain's growth rate might be slow compared to that of other advanced industrial nations. Even if the national income was rising only slowly, yet distributional conflicts about who should get what were blunted. The dividends of growth meant that everyone could get something: both profits and wages could rise, both consumer incomes and public expenditure on the social services could go on increasing. Competition between the Labour and Conservative parties largely revolved around the issue as to which one could successfully lay claim to being the most effective technician of economic growth.

The ever-deepening economic crisis that marked the years after 1973, as growth went into reverse gear, profoundly transformed this situation. The economics of national decline inevitably lead to the politics of conflict: a falling national income meant that competition for ever more scarce resources had become a zero-sum game. While the politics of economic growth had led to convergence between the political parties – both committed to promoting economic growth by means of technocratic planning – the politics of conflict led to an ever-increasing divergence between them. The debate about techniques (means) increasingly turned into a confrontation about ideologies (ends). By the turn of the decade, the Conservative Party, which had been returned to office in 1979, was committed to an ideology of the private market: explicitly repudiating what was perceived to have been the technocratic corporatism of the Heath administration between 1970 and 1974. Conversely, the Labour Party was convulsed by a highly charged ideological debate revolving

around the question of what Socialist principles were and how best
to implement them: a debate marked by the attacks on the managerial corporatism of the 1974 to 1979 Labour administration. The
differences between the two parties had crystallised (to exaggerate
only a little) into a confrontation between the values of individualism
and those of collectivism.

One casualty of the new politics was the faith in technocracy that
had marked the 1960s and early 1970s: the re-politicisation of issues
which had once been defined as belonging properly to the realm of
the expert. If the techniques derived from Keynesian economics
could no longer be relied upon to produce growth, then inevitably
politicians had to handle the conflicts generated by distributional
issues. Moreover, the challenge to expertise was reinforced by a further trend, whose roots lay in the 1960s but which emerged with
ever-increasing visibility in the course of the 1970s.[2] This was the
emphasis on the values of participatory democracy: a revolt against
centralised bureaucracy. Just as successive governments were reorganising the civil service, local government and the health service
on criteria based on the values of efficiency (see previous chapter),
so a groundswell of opposition to these values was making itself felt.
Already in 1968, the publication of the Skeffington report[3] had
reflected the demands for citizen involvement in the processes of
town planning. In the 1970s, the demands increasingly spread to
other policy areas.

The change was reflected in the currency of political rhetoric.
Already in 1974 the Labour manifesto proclaimed that: 'we want to
give a much bigger say to citizens in all their various capacities – as
tenants, shoppers, patients, voters. Or as residents or workers in
areas where development proposals make them feel more planned
against than planned for.' The Conservative manifesto made much
of worker participation in industry and parent participation in the
running of schools.[4] The rhetoric may not have been translated into
action but it was significant as a recognition of a new mood. While
the Right was suspicious of bureaucratic technocracy because of its
individualism, the Left was suspicious because of its commitment
to wider participation in decision-making.

The second half of the 1970s therefore represent a retreat, begun
under the Labour Government and accelerated under the Conservatives, from big government. While political scientists launched the
concept of governmental overload[5] – of an imbalance between the
demands on governments and their capacity to respond – economists
identified rising public expenditure as the source of Britain's eco-

nomic ills.[6] Intellectual arguments apart, in any case, governments had a more direct political incentive to try to restrain public spending: in a period of nil growth, rising public spending meant increasing taxation. Economic crisis compelled a choice between continuing to expand the public sector and maintaining disposable consumer incomes. By 1976 the Labour Government had made its choice. Between 1971–72 and 1975–76, the ratio of public expenditure to national income had risen from 50 to 60 per cent, the 1976 Public Expenditure White Paper pointed out.[7] Now the intention was to reverse this trend, and public expenditure plans were cut accordingly. It was the first of a succession of such attempts to hold back the momentum of the inherited public expenditure policies: attempts which reflected a reluctant concession to economic and political pressures by the Labour Government and an enthusiastic ideological commitment by the Conservative administration.

This, then, was the NHS's new economic, political and intellectual environment in the second half of the 1970s. All the factors identified – the increasing ideological polarisation of politics, the revolt against the values of expertise, the interest in participatory democracy and, above all, the commitment to reducing public expenditure – were to have an influence on the politics of the health care arena, as we shall see. Indeed the internal politics of the health care arena are incomprehensible unless account is taken of these new environmental forces. But, equally, it is important to stress, the process of change was gradual: there was no frontal assault, only a dawning realisation that the perceptions and assumptions which had for so long shaped health care policies required adapting to the new environment.

To a remarkable degree, the NHS remained sheltered, if not insulated, from the harsh new economic and political environment in which it was operating. It was protected, as always, by its continuing popularity. The political consensus – although frayed by ideological battles (see below) – held. In the 1979 election, both parties committed themselves to giving financial priority to the NHS, just as both committed themselves to simplifying its structure. Despite the annual ritual of public expenditure cuts, spending on the NHS was not reduced. In the financial year 1980–81 the current budget of the NHS was £644 million higher in volume terms (measuring the input of real resources), than it had been in 1975–76: a rise of 9.3 per cent over the period.[8] As in the past, and in line with the analysis offered in the previous chapter, successive Secretaries of State traded in reductions in the NHS's investment programme in return for safeguarding the current budget against cuts: capital spending declined throughout the period. In contrast, spending on both education and housing – both programmes which in the 1950s and later had taken precedence over the NHS – actually fell during the same period, substantially so in the case of housing. Clearly, the NHS had moved to the top of the queue in terms of the political priorities in the allocation of resources: its share of the national income was rising (a fact which reflected as much the decline in the national income itself as the increase in the NHS budget).

If the reality was a rising budget, the perception within the NHS was of increasing financial stringency. The rhetoric of financial crisis rose to a crescendo in the second half of the 1970s, and provides the background music to the specific policy issues explored subsequently in this chapter. This is a phenomenon already encountered and explored previously in the context of the 1960s, and many of the factors which explained the perception of inadequacy in a period of expanding budgets in the 1960s continued to be relevant in the 1970s. The demands generated by demographic changes and technological developments continued to assert themselves. Moreover, the gap between what could be done within the budgetary limits of the NHS and would could be done in the health services of wealthier nations widened, if anything, as Britain's national income fell ever further behind that of Sweden, Germany and other advanced industrialised nations.

There were other, more specific reasons. The opening years of the decade had seen an exceptionally fast rate of growth in the NHS budget: an average annual rate of increase of 4.3 per cent under the 1970–74 Conservative Government. In contrast, the equivalent figure under the 1974–79 Labour Government was only 1.5 per cent: the Labour Government's ideological commitment to the NHS having been eroded by the waves of economic crisis.[9] The figure was maintained at the lower level by the incoming Conservative Government in 1979. So, the NHS was a case of relative deprivation over time. Moreover, the perception of stringency was reinforced by growing uncertainty and unpredictability. In 1976 the Treasury introduced a new system for controlling public expenditure: the so-called cash limits system. This meant that if the costs of providing any particular level of public provision rose faster than assumed by the Treasury – particularly if wages and salaries, which accounted for about 70 per cent of the NHS's total budget, increased faster than predicted – there would be no automatic supplementation as in the past. Instead, there would have to be a compensatory cut in the input of real resources. In both 1976–77 and 1979–80, the NHS suffered from a severe cash limits squeeze[10]; all budgetary commitments had to be hurriedly revised during the course of the financial year. In the latter year, there was virtually no growth in the NHS's budget in terms of real resources. The figures of average annual increases thus tend to present a somewhat misleading picture of the NHS's financial position, in so far as they iron out the disconcerting year by year fluctuations.

More important still, financial turbulence threatened to make nonsense of the principles on which the 1974 NHS was designed. The philosophy of reorganisation was, as we have seen, to create an NHS which could carry out rational planning. Reorganisation was followed by a flurry of planning initiatives. In 1976 the DHSS unveiled its planning system: a system whereby the health authorities were intended to produce strategic plans, reflecting DHSS guidelines and national priorities.[11] The same year the DHSS published a priorities document,[12] setting out its objectives for different services: objectives expressed partly in terms of norms of provision and partly in terms of expenditure allocations. At the same time, the department was pursuing its policies for redressing inequities in the geographical distribution of resources by means of differential growth rates in the allocation of funds to the regions. But all these strategies assumed not only growth but some degree of predictability: in other words, the NHS found itself committed to a whole range of policy objectives, forged in the era of optimism about economic prospects, and about the consequent scope for rational long-term planning – just as it entered the era of economic pessimism.

Symbolic of its dilemmas, the NHS found itself increasingly embarrassed by the completion of the hospitals designed and approved in the days of optimism. These had been built on the assumption that future generations would inevitably be better able to afford higher standards than their predecessors; accordingly, their running costs were much higher than those of the buildings they were to replace. Economic crisis had shattered the underlying assumption, but the financial commitments embodied in the new hospitals remained. So the great success story of NHS planning in the 1960s became, ironically enough, one of the causes of financial stringency by the end of the 1970s. It is therefore not surprising (see below) that the faith in planning was, in turn, to become a casualty in the new political and economic environment. Compounding these problems of the NHS, there were the changes within the arena of health care policy: changes which were in part specific to the NHS but which also reflected the wider environmental forces discussed above. It is to an analysis of these that we now turn.

THE EXPLODING HEALTH CARE POLICY ARENA

If the 1960s gave birth to a new spirit of militancy among those working in the NHS, as noted in the previous chapter, by the mid 1970s the infant had grown into a large, aggressive adult. The phenomenon marked the convergence of two trends. While the trade unions began increasingly to demonstrate the kind of obstreperous assertiveness which had once been the monopoly of the medical profession, the medical profession in turn began to use the weapons of industrial warfare which had once been the monopoly of the trade unions. Implicit in this was a shift in the balance of power. For the trade unions – and other organisations representing the non-medical professions in the NHS – militancy was a sign of a growing awareness of their muscle, of their ability to exert pressure by threatening to withdraw their labour. This was a threat which was all the more persuasive given the complex nature of the NHS, and its dependence on the spontaneous co-operation of people with a large variety of skills. In the case of the medical profession, however, militancy reflected a collective sense that power was slipping away from the doctors and towards the other participants in the NHS policy arena: gone were the days when the medical profession could assume that it could get its way without indulging in such unprofessional conduct as taking industrial action.

The growing militancy of the trade unions can be explained partly by reasons specific to the NHS, partly by more general societal factors. For the trade unions, the NHS provided a tempting game reserve for recruitment. Between 1948 and 1974, the proportion of NHS workers belonging to trade unions rose from 40 to 60 per cent, with most of the increase coming in the second half of the period.[13] By the standards of the public sector, however, even 60 per cent represented a low degree of unionisation: in central and local government, the proportion was nearly 90 per cent. So here there was a direct incentive to the trade unions to show their muscle: to advertise the advantages of membership by pressing for higher wages and salaries. The 1973 strike of ancillary workers had not only brought results; it had also destroyed the traditional assumption that people working in the NHS simply did not take industrial action – that their responsibilities to the patients necessarily imposed a self-denying ordinance on them.

Further compounding militancy was the fact the trade unions were competing against each other for members. There were, for example, no clear demarcation lines between the Confederation of Health Service Employees (COHSE) and the National Union of Public Employees (NUPE). The former tended to recruit chiefly among those with the least prestigious professional qualifications, such as the less skilled nurses working in mental care and other long-stay hospitals. The latter tended to recruit chiefly among ancillary workers: hospital porters, ward orderlies and cooks. But there was a considerable degree of overlap between them. Lastly, the trade unions were not only competing against each other but also against professional organisations: in particular, they increasingly challenged the Royal College of Nursing's role of acting both as a professional organisation and as a trade union. Militancy was further encouraged, if only inadvertently, by national policies in the 1970s. It was the National Board for Prices and Incomes which encouraged the introduction of local productivity deals in the NHS, in the hope that pay settlements could become self-financing.[14] Negotiating such deals gave greater salience to the role of the trade unions: an unexpected by-product of the drive for greater national efficiency. Equally important was the recurrent introduction of incomes policies by successive Labour and Conservative governments. These tended to distort traditional patterns of differentials so creating, in time, pressures to restore the inherited wage and salary contours: paradoxically a conservative attachment to inherited patterns thus became a source of radicalism.

The new assertiveness of the NHS workers paid dividends. If the real input of resources into the NHS increased only slowly, the input of money soared up: between 1974 and 1976 alone, there was a rise of 25 per cent in the cost of the NHS (in constant price terms) – reflecting largely a series of expensive pay settlements. Indeed NHS workers did better than the population as a whole.[15] Between 1970 and 1975, the average earnings of British workers rose by 107.8 per cent. The equivalent figure for ancillary workers in the NHS, however, was 134 per cent, while that for nurses was 143 per cent. Only doctors were lagging behind: the equivalent figure for them was 84 per cent.[16]

It is therefore not surprising that the second half of the 1970s was a period of medical militancy, as well as of trade union militancy: of a gradual convergence in the tactics of the trade unions and the professional medical organisations. Medical salaries were particularly affected by incomes policies designed to favour lower-paid

The politics of disillusionment

workers: not only were differentials between doctors and other NHS workers being squeezed, so were differentials within the medical profession. Above all, the medical profession was losing out on the comparability criterion put forward by the 1959 Royal Commission: its earnings were falling behind the comparable professions. The 1976 Review Body report drew attention to the 'anomalies and injustices' created by incomes policy.[17] The 1977 report concluded that the living standards of the average general practitioner or consultant had fallen by 20 per cent between 1975 and 1977.[18] The 1978 report underlined 'the need to reverse the serious decline in morale that has accompanied the decline in pay and standards of living relative to others in comparable walks of life since 1975'.[19] It was not until 1980 that the medical profession collectively managed to re-establish its traditional place in the hierarchy of rewards[20]: a place which was perhaps all the more strongly defended because it reflected the arbitrary accidents of history rather than being based on any rational or objective criteria.

So, for the first time in the history of the NHS, doctors took industrial action. The medical profession collectively had threatened to refuse to co-operate with the Government in both 1911 and 1946. But now, breaking with all precedent, they actually withdrew their labour without withdrawing from the NHS. In October 1975, junior hospital doctors in Leicestershire took industrial action over pay, which subsequently spread to the rest of the country. The details of the dispute are of no concern here.[21] But two aspects of it should be noted. First, contributing to the militancy, there was the competition between the BMA and the Medical Practitioners' Union (which had merged with a trade union, the Association of Scientific, Technical and Managerial Staffs, in 1970): the tactics of the junior doctors largely represented a grassroots revolt against the leadership of the BMA. Second, the outcome of the dispute was the introduction of an industrial-type contract for the junior hospital doctors, with overtime payments for virtually all hours worked over and above the basic 40-hour week: the notion of the professional being someone who looks after his patients at all times of the day and night had taken another knock. In turn, this system of overtime payments led to the erosion of differentials between senior registrars and consultants. The 1977 Review Body report specifically highlighted the consequent 'sense of injustice' felt by consultants.

In any case, the consultants were already embroiled in a battle with the Government over their contracts and private practice (see below). They, too, were adopting militant tactics: their 'sanctions' consisting of threats, only sporadically carried out, to limit their NHS working commitments to care for emergencies only.[22] The threat, made in 1975, split the medical profession. It was publicly criticised by the heads of the Royal Colleges. Even the *British Medical Journal* pointed out that the use of industrial sanctions 'represents a regrettable decline in professional self-esteem which could permanently damage relations between doctors and the public'.[23] The adoption of industrial sanctions would seem to be significant of a profoundly important shift in the position of the medical profession. It eroded the assumption that doctors were somehow different from other workers in the NHS: that their power reflected the legitimate deference paid to a profession with a calling to serve the public – a calling which imposed special responsibilities and inhibitions on them. Sir Theodore Fox, a former editor of *The Lancet* and a much respected medical figure, pointed out that the 'conversion of junior hospital doctors to the methods of militant trade unionism' suggested that 'they are beginning to see themselves as workers in an industry rather than members of a profession – as technologists rather than doctors'.[24]

The divisions within the medical profession ran deep, and in 1977 a special working party representing both the Royal Colleges and the BMA produced a discussion document on the ethical responsibilities of doctors.[25] The report offers an interesting view of how the doctors viewed the implicit concordat between the profession and the Government established in 1946. Doctors, the report conceded, had an ethical responsibility to their patients, but:

Those who maintain that it is always unethical for a professional man to withdraw his services – which in the view of many is the only effective weapon available to him when persuasion fails – are in danger of accepting for doctors a position of subservience to their employers that would preclude them from maintaining their standards. The desire not to harm patients by direct action may then result in harming them by doing nothing. It is unreasonable to expect a profession to remain passive in the face of declining standards, inadequate resources, and lay intervention in the doctor–patient relationship.

It was therefore essential, the report concluded, for

both sides to avoid causes of conflict to a point at which some withdrawal of services becomes the only remedy for doctors to preserve their professional standards and protect the long-term interests of their patients. Government has a special responsibility not to create such conflict by pursuing purely political ends. The profession has a special responsibility not to create such conflict purely to further the advantage of its own members.

The report has been quoted at some length because it shows the nature of the dilemma faced by both government and the medical profession. In a near-monopoly service, each was dependent on the other. Mutual dependence indicated conflict-avoidance strategies: if achieving change in the NHS was difficult, it was because of the inbuilt incentives to seek compromise – and to avoid action on those issues where conflict was inevitable. But since it was the medical profession which determined which policies were being pursued for 'purely political ends', the desire to avoid conflict inevitably tended to reinforce the veto power of the doctors over what appeared on the agenda for discussion.

The report also brings out into the open some of the tensions that were becoming apparent in the health care policy arena in the second half of the 1970s. 'The profession may justifiably think that it has an ethical responsibility to provide the best available treatment', the report argued, 'while the State may regard itself as being responsible to the community to limit the resources available to the National Health Service on criteria other than the needs of the patient.' This conflict was, as previously argued, always implicit in the structure of the NHS, but economic crisis inevitably meant that the other criteria would have greater force. Again, the report's complaint about 'lay intervention in the doctor–patient relationship' reflects the changes that were taking place. For the militancy of the trade unions did not find expression only in battles over pay. At the national level, it led them into a direct conflict with the medical profession over the issue of private beds in NHS hospitals, further discussed below: a direct challenge, as the doctors saw it, to what had hitherto been the medical domain of policy-making. At the local level, trade union members began to assert their right to share in decisions about hospital policy and, more threateningly still, to question clinical judgements. Significantly, it was the trade unions represented in the mental illness and chronic care sector – especially COHSE – which took the lead: this was an area of the NHS where doctors were thin on the ground and where nurses traditionally had played a greater role. In a number of cases, the trade unions challenged medical decisions to admit patients. 'Who was responsible for patients – the consultant or the shop steward?', asked one indignant doctor.[26] In the case of Brookwood Hospital, staff announced the formation of a workers' council to run the 900-bed mental hospital: a significant, albeit temporary, assertion of worker syndicalism in rivalry to medical syndicalism.[27]

Adding to the medical profession's sense of losing control was the growing assertiveness of groups representing NHS consumers. The 1974 reorganisation institutionalised the voice of the consumer, as we have seen, in the shape of Community Health Councils, though their composition betrayed a basic ambiguity as to whether they were supposed to represent the local community as *consumers* of health services or as *citizens*. They were a compromise, as it were, between the demands of consumerism and the demands for participation: the former being essentially a market ideology concerned to maximise value for money and services, the latter being a political ideology concerned to maximise opportunities to influence policy. CHCs varied greatly in their style and their activities.[28] But they not only had the right to demand information; they also had the right to be consulted over decisions to close hospitals and other changes: any decisions not approved by CHCs had to be referred to the DHSS. Their power consisted, as it were, in the ability to throw grit into the normal machinery of NHS decision-making: to impose delays. While CHCs might in some circumstances be seen as allies by the medical profession – as platforms for publicising shortcomings in the service and so reinforcing their demands for more resources – they could also be perceived as a threat: a prime example of 'lay intervention'.

Others, too, were crowding into the health care policy arena. By 1979 a Directory of Organisations for Patients and Disabled People could list over 230 such bodies.[29] Some existed to provide services for deprived groups, to encourage research or to provide information. For example, the aims of the British Migraine Association are to encourage migraine sufferers, to support research and to diffuse information about treatment, while the Sole Mates Club (sic) serves to help 'people with odd shoe sizes to exchange shoes'. Others exist to provide a platform or forum for particular groups of patients or for people with special needs. For example, the Down's Children's Association seeks to 'provide a forum for parents', among other objectives, while the Society To Support Home Confinements aims 'to support, advise and assist women who want a home confinement but meet with difficulties when trying to make the necessary arrangements'. Only a minority of the organisations explicitly give their aim as being to influence policy in the NHS, and thus can be classified as pressure groups in the traditional sense of that versatile phrase. For example, MIND gives its aim as being 'to campaign for the needs and rights of mentally ill and mentally handicapped people', while the British Kidney Patient Association seeks to 'lobby for more facilities'.

The politics of disillusionment

Simply to list some of these organisations is, however, to suggest that even where their aim is not explicitly to exert influence, their mere existence serves to introduce a new factor into the policy-making processes, both nationally and locally. Where previously decisions about maternity care policy were taken by the experts, in the light of their desire to minimise risks and maximise the medical technology available by concentrating all births in specialised hospital centres, now a group exists to articulate the desire of some women to have their babies at home, risks and all. The mere existence of an organisational focus for a particular group of patients is likely to give visibility to their demands. In short, the growth of such organisations multiplies the demands being made on the NHS: demands which may involve calling for the investment of extra resources or which challenge existing clinical and other practices. It is important not to exaggerate. The growth of special interest groups and lobbies should not be interpreted as evidence of a general desire for public involvement in the health care policy arena. For the main characteristics of these groups and lobbies were that they were organised around very specific issues and were run by middle-class activists. Their strength lay precisely in the fact that they were unrepresentative of NHS consumers or citizens at large: that they were exceptionally articulate in putting forward the case for particular interests. But their mere existence represented a question mark against the traditional assumption that health care policies could be determined according to criteria of need and technical excellence, as defined by the experts, as against criteria based on consumer demands. The major battles were still fought out by the big battalions of the health service producers: the theme of the next section. However, the political landscape against which these battles were fought had changed, if only marginally and subtly.

THE POLITICS OF IDEOLOGICAL CONFRONTATION: A CASE STUDY

New forces operating in a new environment inevitably introduced a new kind of politics into the health care policy arena: the politics of ideological confrontation. Between 1974 and 1976 the Labour Government and the medical profession were locked into what was the most bitter political struggle since the inception of the NHS: the battle over private beds. It was not, of course, the first occasion on which the government and the doctors had come into conflict: con-

117

flict over pay, as noted in earlier chapters, provides a recurrent theme running through the entire history of the NHS. The battle over private beds was, however, different in that it threatened the very consensus which in the past had contained conflict. It therefore provides a case study of the impact of the changes in the arena of health care policy, and in its political environment, discussed in the previous section.[30]

The existence of pay beds in NHS hospitals, to which consultants could admit their private fee-paying patients, was a legacy of Bevan's 1946 compromise with the medical profession. They represented a concession to the consultants made in return for their support of the principle of the NHS. In 1974, when the crisis broke, there were 4,500 such pay beds, handling some 120,000 patients a year: they represented just over one per cent of all NHS beds and the private patients treated in them represented two per cent of all non-psychiatric cases handled in the NHS. If pay beds were relatively insignificant in terms of their numbers, however, their symbolic significance to the Labour Party was great. They represented a flaw in the pure crystal of the NHS's underlying conception: the idea that the treatment of patients should be determined exclusively by criteria of need, as distinct from the ability to pay. In theory, pay beds did not affront this principle. Private patients were buying not the right treatment, only the right to be treated by a consultant of their own choice in a room of their own. But in practice, it was argued, pay beds allowed private patients to jump the queue for treatment: there was at least some evidence to suggest that consultants would admit their private patients ahead of other people on the waiting list. The existence of private beds therefore introduced a dual system of standards into the NHS.

The issue was clearly defined by Barbara Castle who became Secretary of State for the Social Services in the incoming Labour Government of 1974, and who led the attack on private beds. 'The issue before us is whether the facilities of the NHS, which are supposed to be available only on the principle of medical priority, should contain facilities that are available on the different principle of ability to pay. We say that those two principles are incompatible in the NHS', she told Parliament in 1974. In other words, the issue was central to Labour's vision of itself as a crusader for social justice. The religious metaphor is apt, as Mrs Castle was to point out on a subsequent occasion: 'Intrinsically the National Health Service is a church. It is the nearest thing to the embodiment of the Good Samaritan that we have in any respect of our public policy. What

would we say of a person who argued that he could only serve God
properly if he had pay pews in his church?' *Barbara Castle*

Given this fundamental incompatability between Labour's vision
of the NHS and the existence of private beds, the decision to tackle
this issue may seem the inevitable outcome of a long-standing ideological commitment. Barbara Castle was simply paying an overdue
political debt to the party's ideals. But this still leaves an unex-
plained puzzle. Labour's hostility to private beds was long-standing.
But the previous Labour Government, in office from 1964 to 1970,
had done nothing about them. Kenneth Robinson, the Labour Minister of Health, had reduced the number of pay beds, not on ideological grounds but because they were much under-utilised: he did
so in agreement with the medical profession, in return for lifting the
limits on the fees that could be charged by consultants. So why did
the 1974 Labour Government act, while its predecessor had reso-
lutely ignored the issue?

One explanation lies in the increasing salience of the issue within
the Labour Party. In 1971 the Labour majority on the Employment
and Social Services Sub-Committee of the Parliamentary Expenditure Committee exploited an inquiry into NHS facilities for private
patients to direct attention to the abuse (as they saw it) of these
facilities. Their report argued that the system of pay beds permitted
'queue jumping for non-medical reasons', that it was unfair on junior
hospital doctors, nurses and technicians 'used for private purposes
and without willing consent', and that it encouraged consultants to
congregate in those parts of the country where there was greatest
scope for private practice. The report was based on thin evidence,
but its conclusions had resonance within the Labour Party. The
Party's latent sensitivity on this issue was activated. The 1974
Labour manifesto pledged the Party to 'phase out private practice
from the hospital service'. The manifesto also pledged the Labour
Party to carry out another long-standing ideological commitment:
to 'abolish prescription charges'. This, however, remained a dead-
letter throughout the Labour Government's period in office. So the
implementation of the pledge to phase out private beds cannot be
seen as the inevitable consequence of the manifesto commitment.
There was nothing automatic about the implementation of such
pledges, particularly if they cost money. Barbara Castle's decision
to act on the issue of pay beds reflected the changing balance of
power both within the health care policy arena and in its environment. The political costs of doing nothing had become greater than
the political costs of action.

No sooner was Barbara Castle installed in office, than her hand was forced. At Charing Cross Hospital – one of London's major teaching hospitals, strategically situated for attracting the attention of the media – members of NUPE took strike action in an attempt to force the closure of the private wing. Sporadically, similar action followed in other hospitals throughout the country: action which perhaps reflected as much hostility to the special privileges enjoyed by private patients, and the extra income derived by consultants, as ideological commitment. Barbara Castle tried to enlist the support of the trade union leaders to head off this attempt to take direct action. But as Len Murray, the Secretary-General of the Trades Union Congress told her, 'Congress is in favour of getting rid of private practice'.[31] Although the leaders of the health service trade unions had not instigated the industrial action – 'we didn't spark off the campaign . . . the issue blew up fortuitously', one of them remarked – the strikes had given political visibility to their own, long-standing commitment to closing private beds. Even if they had wanted to do so, they could not now consign this commitment to the limbo of pledges made in the confident belief that they would never have to be implemented. Nor could the Labour Government, dependent as it was on the co-operation of the trade unions for the success of its economic policies. While it might have been able to ride out the protests of the grassroots movement, it could not afford to ignore the demands of organised labour: private beds would be phased out.

The attack on private beds was essentially ideological: an attack on visible symbols of privilege. But the more general issue of private practice also raised some non-ideological issues. If private practice was obnoxious in principle to the Labour Party, it was irritating in practice to those committed to introducing more rational planning in the NHS. By the mid-1970s, the proportion of consultants holding part-time contracts – that is, ones permitting them to engage in private practice – had fallen to below 50 per cent. But the very existence of the system introduced some perverse incentives into the NHS. While the aim of public policy was to encourage the development of the mental illness, geriatric and chronic care services, part-time contracts gave doctors an incentive to move into those specialties where the opportunities for private practice were greatest. Thus 94 per cent of all consultants in geriatric medicine had whole-time contracts, as against less than 15 per cent in general surgery. Similarly, while the aim of public policy was to achieve a better geographical distribution of specialists and other doctors, part-time contracts gave doctors an incentive (as the Expenditure Committee had noted) to move into those parts of the country where opportunities for private practice were greatest, notably London and other well-provided regions.

At the same time that Barbara Castle was pursuing the issue of pay beds, the Minister of Health – Dr David Owen, who could by no stretch of the imagination be described as a left-wing ideologue – was therefore trying to negotiate a new contract with the consultants. These negotiations had begun in 1972: the consultants, fired by the success of the general practitioners and junior hospital doctors, were themselves anxious to negotiate a new form of contract. In particular, they wanted to secure a contract where payments would be more directly related to the amount of work done: where their commitments to the NHS would no longer be open-ended and where, consequently, they would have a chance to supplement their basic salaries by overtime and other payments. But the Labour Government introduced a new element into the negotiations. It sought to introduce financial incentives designed to encourage full-time practice in the NHS. Extra rewards were to go to those consultants who committed themselves wholly to the NHS; the merit award system, which tended to be biased towards the most prestigious specialties where private practice flourished, was to be replaced by payments for particularly valuable contributions to the running of the service – payments available only to whole-timers, moreover.

The combination of the Labour Government's commitment to phasing out pay beds from the NHS and of the new proposals for loading the consultant contract in favour of full-time consultants turned out to be explosive. For the medical profession, these steps represented a repudiation of the 1946 concordat: an attempt by the Labour administration to abolish the right of doctors to engage in private practice. No matter that Barbara Castle assured them that she merely wanted to separate private practice from the NHS, not to abolish it; the suspicions of the doctors were reinforced by the 1975 Labour Party Conference which voted, much to Barbara Castle's dismay, in favour of the outright abolition of all private medicine. No matter that a majority of consultants, the full-timers, would actually benefit from the proposed changes in the contract: even if the leaders of the profession had been disposed to compromise, the rivalry between the BMA and the Hospital Consultants' and Specialists' Association meant that they were engaged in a competition in militancy.

For the medical profession, as for the Labour Party, the issue of private practice was symbolic. Self-interest was, of course, involved. Private practice added on average something like 20 per cent to the incomes of those NHS consultants who engaged in it. Moreover, a minority of consultants could make much more: one indignant consultant, appalled at the prospect of losing his pay beds, pointed out that he could double his NHS income simply by carrying out 24 private operations a year.[32] More centrally, any threat to private practice aroused the medical profession's fear of total dependancy on the State. If many consultants and other doctors who did not benefit personally from private practice yet fought to preserve it, the reason was that it was a symbol of professional independence. It was, in truth, a fragile symbol. The reality was that doctors did depend financially on the State, and that private practice represented not an alternative to their incomes from the NHS but icing on the cake. But perhaps it was the very fragility of the symbol that made doctors all the more sensitive to perceived threats. The confrontation that followed between Ministers and the medical profession was more bitter than any in the history of the NHS. Nothing like it had been seen since the days when Bevan was embattled with the general practitioners. Meetings between Ministers and the medical profession inevitably ended in acrimony, as Mrs Castle faithfully recorded in her diaries. Finally, the medical profession, as noted in the previous section, mobilised for battle: its ultimate deterrent – sanctions – was wheeled on stage.

Like other ultimate deterrents, that of the medical profession was more for show than use. In any case, as we have already seen, doctors were by no means unanimous in supporting such a weapon. Similarly, the Government did not want to risk an all-out battle with the medical profession. 'This Cabinet had no fire in its belly for this particular fight', Barbara Castle noted at one point in the negotiations.[33] Moreover, within the DHSS, civil servants were unenthusiastic in their support for their Minister's policies. From their point of view, the long-term political costs of a confrontation with the medical profession over the issue of private practice outweighed any possible benefits. If Barbara Castle was dependent on the support of her political constituency in the Labour Party and the trade unions, her civil servants were dependent on the organisational constituency of the NHS. Phasing out private beds might well be desirable; negotiating a new contract might well be advantageous. But maintaining a working relationship with the medical profession was essential if other desirable or advantageous aims of policy were to be achieved in future. There was no point in exhausting the capital

of goodwill over a largely symbolic issue. Not surprisingly, therefore, moves to devise a compromise soon followed. In 1975 Harold
Wilson, the Prime Minister, intervened. He brought into action
Lord Goodman, an experienced mediator, to act as go-between
between Barbara Castle and the medical profession over the issue of
pay beds. He also set up a Royal Commission to examine the state
of the NHS: so responding to the demands of the doctors for an
inquiry into the whole basis, financial as well as organisational, of
the NHS.

The Goodman compromise, translated into legislation in 1976
with virtually no changes, was based on two principles. First, it was
agreed that private beds and facilities should be separated from the
NHS. Second, the Government formally recognised that private
practice should be maintained in Britain, and that doctors should
be entitled to work both privately and in NHS establishments. All
this was in line with Mrs Castle's own Consultative Document on
Private Practice published in 1975.[34] But the Goodman formula
included other features designed to reassure the medical profession.
Only one thousand of the pay beds were to be phased out immediately. Decisions about phasing out the rest were to be taken not
by the Secretary of State but by an independent board with half its
four members drawn from the medical profession and the rest
appointed after consultations with the trade unions and other interested parties; an independent chairman would have the casting vote.
The board, to quote the Secretary of State, would be guided by the
following criteria in phasing out pay beds: 'That there should be a
reasonable demand for private medicine in the area of the country
served by a particular hospital; that sufficient accommodation and
facilities existed in the area for the reasonable operation of private
medicine, and that all reasonable steps had been, or were being
taken to provide those alternative beds and facilities.' In contrast to
the Consultative Document, which had proposed that the total size
of the private sector should be frozen, no such limit was set under
the Goodman formula. Similarly, no date was set for the completion
of the phasing out operation. In 1980 – when the Health Services
Board, set up to implement these policies, was wound up by the
Conservative Government – the number of pay beds in England had
been reduced from 3,444 to 2,533.[35]

The negotiations over the consultant contract dragged on for the
remainder of the Labour Government's term of office. Again, the
outcome was a compromise. The profession secured changes
designed to 'relate remuneration more closely to the work done'[36]:

in other words, consultants were to share in the opportunities, already enjoyed by their juniors, to get overtime payments. In exchange, the DHSS obtained changes which slightly tilted the financial advantage towards full-time consultants. The proposal to abolish the merit award system was dropped; in return, though, it also was to be amended to favour full-timers. However, the 1979 contract never came into force. Disagreement about its pricing – not about its principles – prevented its implementation. It was left to the incoming Conservative Government to introduce a new contract (see below).

In the end, therefore, the consensus about the NHS emerged from the post-1974 crises battered and frayed but still basically intact. Conflict had, after all, been constrained by consensus. In retrospect the bitterness aroused by the issues involved seemed disproportionate to their importance. As the Royal Commission put it in its 1979 report, 'We have reached no conclusions about the overall balance of advantage or disadvantage of the existence of a private sector . . . but it is clear that whichever way it lies it is small as matters now stand'. Moreover, it pointed out, 'From the point of view of the NHS the main importance of pay beds lies in the passions aroused'.[37]

If the drama of these years did little to change the nature of the NHS, it did, however, illuminate the changed nature of the health care policy arena itself. Not only did the issue of pay beds represent a threat to the existing order – the intrusion of political ideology into the NHS's organisational ideology, with its emphasis on incremental change achieved through consensus-engineering – but it also revealed powerful new actors on stage: the trade unions. It showed that, in the last resort, the medical profession could only respond to the challenge of these new forces by adopting their tactics and by conceding openly that its own power rested not on its professional status but on its ability to use its industrial muscle.

THE POLITICS OF ORGANISATIONAL STASIS

The confrontation between the medical profession and the Government, the growing assertiveness of the trade unions and the gradual tightening of the NHS's budget all contributed to the sense of crisis which marked the second half of the 1970s. 'We were appointed at a time when there was widespread concern about the NHS', the Royal Commission commented in its 1979 report. Not for the first time the NHS offered the seemingly paradoxical spectacle of contented consumers and disgruntled producers. While the consumers were continuing to show overwhelming satisfaction with the services provided by the NHS, as shown by surveys carried out on behalf of the Royal Commission,[38] the producers were protesting about falling standards. If there was a revolution of frustrated expectations, it was among the producers not among the consumers.

To an extent the discontent of the producers – doctors, nurses and others – reflected a special characteristic of the NHS discussed earlier: the fact that producers had a direct incentive to emphasise the shortcomings of the NHS in order to dramatise their own case for better pay and conditions of work. But compounding this endemic discontent was the dry rot of disillusionment with the new structure of the NHS created by the 1974 reorganisation. This disillusionment was, to a large extent perhaps, merely the rationalisation of a general sense of frustration reflecting the gap between the hopes aroused in the years of optimism and the financial reality of the years of economic crisis. But it also reflected the fact that the reorganised NHS was not delivering the goods: that the vision of a rationally planned health service was not being translated into reality. On the contrary, the reorganised NHS appeared to have introduced new obstacles in the way of implementing change.

Hardly had the new NHS been inaugurated, than the critics of Sir Keith Joseph's architecture appeared to have been justified. The new structure, it was widely agreed, was indeed too complex. Designed to please everyone, the structure satisfied no one. By 1977 a survey of 482 administrators and others working in the NHS[39] showed overwhelming dissatisfaction with the structure. Four-fifths of those interviewed favoured some change to reduce the number of tiers. Moreover, structural complexity did lead to greater bureaucracy – at least as measured by the number of administrators employed. The number of administrative and clerical staff rose from 87,000 in 1973 to 113,000 in 1976, when the DHSS launched a drive to cut the costs of management. Nor, on the face of it, had the new NHS solved the problems which it was designed to tackle. Implicit in the reorganisation was a clear separation in the functions of central government and the peripheral health authorities, encapsulated in the gnomic phrase (quoted in Ch. 3) of 'maximum delegation downward, maximum accountability upward'. The centre would lay down policy objectives; the periphery would implement them. In practice reorganisation did little to resolve the tensions between centre and periphery, inherent in the concept of the NHS as a national service financed out of public funds.

For how could the DHSS delegate, while it remained accountable to Parliament for every penny spent? Not surprisingly, the complaints about excessive interference by the centre that followed organisation were remarkably similar to those already encountered in the pre-organisation days. In 1976 a report produced by the chairmen of the regional authorities[40] rehearsed a familiar litany of grievances. The DHSS was exercising an excessive degree of control over building: 'Rather than promote the economic and effective use of capital, the system of detailed checking produces interference in minutiae and certainly results in duplication of staff and effort; there is often argument over petty design detail, and above all lengthy delay.' Moreover, the department – in the view of the regional chairmen – spent an excessive amount of time following up the three thousand parliamentary questions that were asked every year by MPs: the DHSS should leave it to the field authorities to deal with these questions and resist the temptation 'to interpret or check the results'. Overall, those working in the NHS were baffled by the complexity of the DHSS's internal structure, frustrated by the department's habit of 'proffering advice on unattainable objectives which cannot be funded' and resentful of the rigidity imposed by national agreements about numbers of staff and levels of pay: 'Too often in the NHS, authorities are forced under existing regulations to employ staff of inadequate calibre, where fewer – but better – people would produce much more effective results.' And the report concluded by calling for 'A reduction in the functions performed by the DHSS and a consequent reduction in size'. The department's chief function should be to act 'as the midwife of ideas' – leaving detailed implementation to the administrators and professionals at the periphery who, in any case, were better informed and better equipped than the rotating cast of civil servants at the centre to take decisions.

Yet while those at the periphery were voicing their resentment of central control, Parliament was voicing its dissatisfaction at the lack of effective accountability. The Committee of Public Accounts was pressing the DHSS to tighten up financial control: 'We remain disturbed about the effectiveness of the financial control exercised by some health authorities, and we recommend that urgent consideration should continue to be given to means of improving financial control and accountability within the present structure', it reported in 1977.[41] The Social Services Sub-Committee of the Expenditure Committee was urging the DHSS to devise more effective tools for monitoring what was happening in the NHS. Expenditure statistics, it argued in 1977, should be complemented by information about 'the adequacy or otherwise of the services provided, in terms either of the availability of facilities for treatment or of standards of care'.[42] The theme was to recur, again and again, in the reports of the Expenditure Committee's successor, the Social Services Committee. Its 1980 report, for example, stressed the need to develop 'a comprehensive information system which would permit this Committee and the public to assess the effects of changes in expenditure levels or patterns on the quality and scope of services provided'.[43]

The DHSS's dilemma – caught in a crossfire of criticism from both the NHS authorities and Parliament – further underlines a fundamental weakness in the whole concept of rational planning which underlay reorganisation. The rhetoric was all about accountability and monitoring. But what was the currency of accountability and where were the tools of monitoring? It was easy enough to establish a machinery of financial accountability and an administrative hierarchy responsible for monitoring. But it was much more difficult to answer questions about what the money was buying in terms of services provided to patients or about the quality of the care being offered. The required instruments of measurement simply did not exist. Indeed the available information was dangerously ambiguous. The DHSS might well have figures of the unit costs of treating patients in acute beds or patients in hospitals for the mentally handicapped. The general presumption was that it was desirable to lower the unit costs of treating each acute patient (since this was a sign of increased efficiency) and to increase the unit costs of caring for long-stay patients (since this was a sign of improved quality as measured by the input of staff). This, indeed, was the aim of DHSS policy, and by the end of the 1970s, it was succeeding.[44] But there remained some nagging questions. What if lower unit costs in acute beds reflected, as the doctors were inclined to claim, not increased efficiency but lower quality? What if higher unit costs in the chronic care sector reflected not better quality care for patients but more leisure for staff?

In the attempt to answer such questions, the DHSS inevitably was drawn into taking a close interest in the implementation of policy. The only information available was qualitative, DHSS witnesses repeatedly told the Social Services Committee: the impressions of the department's professionals. Only professionals, in other words, could assess the work of other professionals. Judgements of adequacy or quality could not be derived from statistics but had to be based on expert opinion. Much the same was true of planning. The DHSS might publish priorities documents setting out desirable

127

objectives expressed in norms of inputs (whether beds or nurses) for particular client groups such as the mentally handicapped or the elderly. Similarly, the department might publish a programme budget showing the desired shifts in expenditure patterns as between different client groups. But, given the principle of infinite diversity, the department could not impose such norms irrespective of local circumstances. On closer inspection, the DHSS's apparently solid policy targets dissolved under the acid of reservations. 'Local priorities will naturally be affected by a range of factors – demographic, social and practical – peculiar to individual areas; and it is accepted that local plans will often not correspond to the order of national priorities proposed here', the DHSS's 1976 Priorities Document admitted. And its 1977 successor made it clear that the expenditure objectives – envisaging a shift of resources to favour the elderly and other deprived groups, and from the hospital to the community services – were 'not specific targets to be reached by declared dates in any locality'.[45] In practice the language of norms and objectives turned out to be merely a vocabulary of exhortation.

No wonder that studies of policy-making within individual health authorities have unanimously come to the conclusion that national priorities impinged at best marginally on local decision-making: that decisions were shaped, unsurprisingly, by the constraints of inherited commitments and the balance of power within the arena of local health care policy.[46] Exhortation could help to nudge such decisions in the direction desired by the central department; for example, between 1975–76 and 1979–80 the average annual expenditure on geriatric services rose by 2.3 per cent, as against only 1.1 per cent for acute services, while spending on community services rose marginally faster than that on hospital services.[47] The price to be paid for such success was, once again, continued pressure and intervention by the DHSS. If planning could not be carried out in terms of imposing centrally determined norms and standards on the periphery, then it inevitably became a process of negotiation between the two sides. If rationality was not to be found in *techniques* – by devising formulas for priorities and standards on the basis of consulting the entrails of epidemiological statistics or the application of other scientific methods – then it had to be sought in *process*: in institutionalising dialogue between centre and periphery. In short, the experience of attempting to plan rationally not only led to greater scepticism about the concept itself, as awareness of the technical problems involved grew,[48] but also perpetuated the dominating role of the DHSS. If the rationality of any policy had to be tested by the way in which it was implemented locally, then the DHSS could not disinterest itself. Contrary to the hopeful assumptions made before 1974, the line between policy-making and implementation was far too blurred to permit a neat separation of central and local functions.

The years following 1974 also undermined some of the other assumptions underlying the 1974 reorganisation. The justification for introducing an area tier into the administrative structure of the NHS was, it will be recalled, that co-terminosity between health and local authorities would lead to co-operation. Experience suggested otherwise,[49] even though in 1976 the DHSS introduced financial incentives designed to encourage collaboration: ear-marked grants for schemes jointly worked out between health and local authorities. Predictably the incentives built into the very structure of the two services turned out to be stronger: each of the two services had an incentive to off-load problems on to the other, each tended to define issues in terms of the rather different perspectives of its own professionals. Moreover, government policies – while extolling the virtues of co-operation at the local level – were themselves notably lacking in co-ordination at the national level. If the DHSS was anxious to encourage the development of community services, the Treasury was even more anxious to cut back the growth of local government spending. Even while the DHSS was planning on the assumption of expansions in such local government services, the Treasury was making it impossible. From 1979 onward the Government was putting pressure on local authorities to cut spending on the personal social services.[50]

Again, the architects of the 1974 reorganisation had assumed that defining the roles of the members of the new Area Health Authorities more tightly would produce more effective management. Not only would members of AHAs be collectively accountable for implementing national policy, but they, in turn, would also ensure that their officers were accountable to them. In practice, AHA members turned out to be a weak link in the chain of accountability. On the one hand, according to a 1977 survey,[51] they 'found it difficult because of lack of time as much as of knowledge to come to grips with so complex a system'. On the other hand, the consensus system of decision-making in officer teams meant that AHA members tended to be offered agreed solutions, not alternative proposals, so giving them little scope to influence policy. The gap between the role accorded to AHAs in the philosophy of reorganisation and their actual performance, between the doctrine and the practice of accountability, is admirably illustrated by the example of the Normansfield Hospital Inquiry[52]: a case study which also illuminates some of the other themes developed in this chapter. The inquiry was held in 1978, nine years after the similar inquiry into conditions at Ely (see previous chapter), which had illustrated many of the weaknesses in the pre-reorganisation NHS and reinforced the case for changes. Like Ely, Normansfield was a hospital for the mentally handicapped. Like the Ely inquiry, the Normansfield inquiry revealed some scandalous conditions.

Perhaps the most significant aspect of the Normansfield affair – as revealed in the inquiry – was that everyone had known about the problems that afflicted the hospital. Everybody, at all levels, was well aware that 'the standard of nursing care was extremely low and the quality of life of many of the patients suffered accordingly'. Everybody, too, knew the main cause: the personal eccentricities and conduct of the consultant psychiatrist whose running battle with nursing staff and medical colleagues turned the familiar problems of hospitals for the mentally handicapped, decaying buildings and staff shortages, into what one visitor described as a 'time-bomb'. The CHC had done its duty by protesting about conditions at Normansfield. A succession of visitors – from the DHSS, from the region and from the AHA – agreed that the situation was appalling. But nothing was done, until a strike by the nurses compelled the setting up of the inquiry, which in turn eventually led to the retirement of the consultant.

A number of significant implications flow from this episode. First, it once again shows the new militancy of the NHS workers. Second, it demonstrates the limits to CHC influence: CHCs could protest, but they could not compel action. Third, it underlines the ineffectiveness of AHA members. 'The conditions we saw during our four days of visiting', the inquiry report commented, 'gave every appearance of being of some duration and were such as to make us wonder how sensitive, caring members of the Authority could have tolerated them without vigorous protest leading to concerted action by officials of the Authority.' Fourth, it suggests that both the central department and the regional authority were prepared to invoke the doctrine of delegation of responsibility in order to avoid being drawn into a messy imbroglio. Lastly, and perhaps most important, it demonstrates the importance of the inertia factor in the NHS as a whole: the difficulty of introducing change – in particular when change involved dealing with a consultant.

The paradox of the reorganised NHS was that it strengthened the inertia factor at precisely the point – as argued at the beginning

of this chapter – in the history of the service when external pressures and internal demands were reinforcing the need for change. If
new priorities to favour the deprived groups of patients were to be
implemented in a period of only marginal growth in the total NHS
budget, then this could only be achieved by shifting resources from
existing services. If geographical equity in the distribution of
resources was to be achieved, then once again resources would have
to be shifted from the well-endowed to the poorly endowed parts of
the country. The latter problem was particularly acute at the sub-
regional level. The national formula for allocating resources to the
regions – the RAWP formula – did not involve cutting the funds of
any region. If the rate of differential growth slowed down, and the
date for achieving equity kept on being postponed, at least all the
regions could count on getting at least a marginal increment every
year. But within the regions things were different, particularly in
the case of London. In the national context, the London regions
were relatively over-provided. But within them, many of the areas
were under-provided. While the population of London was mobile,
hospitals were not; while the population moved into the suburbs,
and beyond, inner London was left with an embarrassing surplus
of hospitals. The demands of the outer London areas could only be
satisfied by cutting hospital provision in inner London: demands
which were all the more insistent since the creation of AHAs had
given political visibility to the distribution of resources below the
regional level.[53]

Reorganisation had, however, increased the costs of such adaptation by institutionalising the right to oppose change. The ability
to veto change – or, at the very least, to resist it by imposing delays
– had been diffused. Within the NHS, any decision had to go
through the elaborate system of advisory committees which had been
set up in 1974. Outside the NHS, a variety of other bodies also had
to be consulted: the emphasis on co-ordinating health and local
authority services inevitably led to the perfectly logical conclusion
that NHS planning should no longer be an introspective process.
Thus the DHSS handbook on planning instructed AHAs to consult:
CHCs, local authorities, the Family Practitioner Committee, the
various Area Advisory Committees and the Joint Staff Consultative
Committee. In addition to the formal mechanisms introduced by the
1974 reorganisation, however, the expansion of the health care policy arena reinforced the opposition to change. No sooner was a hospital threatened by closure then informal action committees sprang
up: coalitions of workers whose jobs were threatened and groups of

citizens whose access to their local health facilities was in danger. If national policy was designed to bring about equity, local interests had an interest in perpetuating inequity where the existing distribution of resources favoured them.

The point is well illustrated by a case history drawn from the research evidence submitted to the Royal Commission[54]: the closure of Poplar Hospital – a small institution, built in 1855, in the East End of London. The dispute over the closure started in 1972; the doors of the hospital did not actually close until the end of 1975. It is a reminder therefore that while the reorganisation of the NHS may have exacerbated the problems of change, the new structure cannot be blamed for all the difficulties. The most significant aspect of the long-drawn-out process was the militancy and numbers of the local opposition groups. Just taking this one local health care policy arena, the actors included: consultants, the Hospital's League of Friends, local MPs, the local Labour Party, a specially formed Save Poplar Campaign, NUPE, local councillors and the Transport and General Workers' Union. The strategy of delay included both a local press campaign and appeals to the Secretary of State. The issue moved repeatedly up and down the decision-making hierarchy: from the District Management Team to the Area, from the Area to the Region, from the Region to the DHSS, and so *da capo*. The wonder is not that it took three years to close Poplar Hospital but that it was ever closed at all.

To describe the delays and administrative costs involved in implementing change may, however, understate the full effect of the growing capacity of an increasing number of actors to throw grit into the machinery: to introduce politics into the self-contained world of the NHS and to challenge the monopoly of technical expertise in decision-making. This could only be measured in terms of the decisions that were not even contemplated for fear of the consequences: the way in which the new political and organisational factors constrained the sense of what was feasible. If the emphasis on decision-making through agreement – the hallmark of the 1974 reorganisation – had started out as a strategy for mobilising consent to change, it had ended up as a strategy for encouraging the mobilisation of opposition to change. The perverse irony, it turned out, was that public interest in health care policy seemed to be a function of opposition to national policies. Once again we recognise a familiar phenomenon in health care politics: while national constituencies for change are diffuse, local constituencies representing the *status quo* are concentrated and organised. It was a phenomenon which

contributed in no small measure to the sense of disillusionment
with the possibilities for using the NHS as an instrument of rational
social engineering that characterised the late 1970s.

BACK TO THE DRAWING BOARD: THE CONSENSUS UNDER
CHALLENGE

The report of the Royal Commission on the NHS, published in
1979, both reflected the growing disillusionment and represented an
attempt to maintain the consensus. It accepted the need for a simplification in the structure of the NHS: thus adding its seal of
approval to the new conventional wisdom that there was one tier too
many. But it reaffirmed the basic philosophy of the NHS. Like the
1956 Guillebaud report, it argued that there was no way of settling
the argument as to what the appropriate level of financing for the
NHS was: the 'right', level of spending was essentially a metaphysical concept. Moreover, it pointed out that 'international comparisons do not suggest that greater expenditure automatically leads to
better health . . . and it is at least arguable that the improvement
in the health of the nation would be greater if extra resources were,
for example, devoted to better housing'. The Royal Commission
therefore rejected the notion that a change in the method of financing health services, such as adopting an insurance-based system,
would solve the problems of the NHS. Like the Guillebaud Committee, too, the Royal Commission conceded the attractions in principle of transferring responsibility for health services to local
government, but rejected it on grounds of feasibility – not least
because such a solution would be unacceptable to the NHS producers, the trade unions among them.

   This is not to suggest that the Royal Commission's report simply
represented a blessing of the *status quo*. In all, its report made 117
recommendations. Some indeed were radical. For example, it proposed that Family Practitioner Committees should be abolished and
their functions assumed by health authorities, in order to incorporate general practice into the mainstream of the NHS. Again, in an
attempt to resolve the conflict between centre and periphery, it proposed that the regional health authorities should be directly accountable to Parliament for the delivery of services, while the DHSS
would only be accountable for national policies. But, overall, its
report was an overwhelming – though not uncritical – endorsement
of the NHS's achievements. In this respect it again resembled the

Guillebaud report. But while the Guillebaud report virtually silenced political argument about the NHS for ten years, that of the Royal Commission marked on the contrary the beginning of a new debate. For while the Royal Commission had been set up by a Labour Government to reassure medical and public opinion, in the hope that it would defend the consensus against criticism, its report was published only three months before the installation of a Conservative Government in office. If the incoming Labour Government of 1974 had brought its own ideological commitments in its luggage, so did the incoming Conservative administration of 1979. The 1979 Conservative administration, in strong contrast to its 1970 predecessor, was not committed to the ideology of rational planning. On the contrary, as noted at the beginning of this chapter, it explicitly repudiated this ideology. Instead, it invoked the virtues of minimal government and the market economy.

Inevitably these themes were reflected – if only in a subdued, minor key – in its policies for the NHS. 'We will simplify and decentralise the service and cut back bureaucracy', the Party's 1979 manifesto proclaimed. While the rhetoric of decentralisation and hostility to bureaucracy were by 1979 the common language of political debate about the NHS, reflecting general disillusionment with the paternalistic rationalisers, the Conservative manifesto also promised to end 'Labour's vendetta against the private health sector'. Lastly, the manifesto raised the possibility, no more, of long-term changes in the methods of funding the NHS.

In the event, Patrick Jenkin, the new Conservative Secretary of State, carried out the manifesto's specific commitments.[55] Labour's policies towards private practice were smartly reversed: an act of ideological restitution, as it were. The policy of phasing out pay beds was abandoned; the Health Services Board was scrapped. Tax relief on medical insurance schemes operated by employers was restored. Finally, a new contract was quickly negotiated with the consultants. This permitted all consultants to engage in some private practice without loss of earnings, while the differentials between part-timers and full-timers was narrowed. In this respect, tactical considerations reinforced ideological bias. Given that demands for extra resources for the NHS tend to come from concentrated and organised labour within the service rather than from diffuse and unorganised patients outside it, then a Government concerned to limit public spending (as the 1979 Conservative administration was) may find it cheaper to buy off the producers than to try to satisfy the consumers. Investment in silencing consultants, and other interest groups within the

The politics of disillusionment

NHS, may thus be seen as an alternative strategy to expanding the service as a whole. In return for the new contract the consultants further agreed to self-policed guidelines designed to prevent queue-jumping by their private patients.

Similarly, if less controversially, the new Conservative Ministers carried out their manifesto pledge to decentralise the NHS. Their proposals faithfully reflected the change in opinion that had taken place since 1974, which is well caught in the following two quotations:

> In the reorganised service, there will be a more systematic and comprehensive planning process than now exists. The Department will annually prepare guidance on national policy objectives for AHAs and RHAs who will then draw up their plans for the development of their services to meet these objectives together with their own local priorities . . . The reorganisation of the Department will provide for it to have close and more regular contact than in the past with the health authorities . . .

> We are determined to see that as many decisions as possible are taken at the local level – in the hospital and in the community. We are determined to have more local health authorities, whose members will be encouraged to manage the Service, with the minimum of interference by any central authority, whether at region or in central government departments.

The first quotation comes from the 1972 White Paper on reorganisation published by the then Conservative Secretary of State, Sir Keith Joseph. The second quotation comes from the Consultative Document on reorganisation, *Patients First*, published by Patrick Jenkin in December 1979,[56] and subsequently incorporated, with only minor modifications, in the legislation and consequential regulations which shaped the new NHS unveiled in 1982.

The central feature of the 1982 model NHS was the simplification of the NHS structure: the central tier – the AHAs – disappeared. These were replaced by District Health Authorities (DHAs). As in the years leading up to 1948, and again up to 1974, there was some debate about the role of the regional authorities. But, in the outcome, the regions were reprieved. While the Government rejected outright the proposal of the Royal Commission for a strengthened regional role – on the grounds that direct regional accountability to Parliament would be incompatible with the Secretary of State's responsibilities for the NHS as a whole – a review of the RHAs was relegated to the indefinite future. If anything the logic of replacing 90 AHAs by some 200 DHAs, a change which inevitably compounds the problems of control by the DHSS, would suggest a strengthened regional role in future.

The central role of the new District Health Authorities in the new model NHS reflected the change in the 'public philosophy' that had taken place during the 1970s and that was complete by the 1980s. Where the 1974 reorganisation emphasised the values of efficiency and rationality (see the quotation from Sir Keith Joseph's White Paper, above) the 1982 reorganisation stressed the virtues of localism and small size. 'The thrust of our policy', one of the DHSS Ministers, Sir George Younger, told Parliament, 'is to have decisions taken as near to the point of delivery of services as is possible.' The DHAs should be established, a government circular laid down,[57] 'for the smallest possible geographical areas within which it is possible to carry out the integrated planning, provision and development' of health services. Only in the most exceptional cases would Ministers permit DHAs to have a population of more than 500,000 or less than 150,000. In the event, these instructions were carried out somewhat flexibly, influenced seemingly by local political pressures[58]; one DHA has a population of over 800,000, while a handful have populations below 100,000.

One criticism made of the change was that it would dilute the scarce resources of technical expertise available in the NHS. Before 1974 the relevant specialists in community medicine, statistics and planning were concentrated at the AHA level, and even so were in short supply. Now, in the remodelled NHS, they are scattered more thinly still, with the DHAs under pressure to cut the costs of management. But this criticism misses the whole point of the 1982 reorganisation, in so far as it represents a revolt against expertise. Given the underlying assumption that local people know best, there was inevitably less scope for the expert. Appropriately enough, Conservative Ministers repudiated the great technological dream of the 1960s – the giant District General Hospital – at the same time as they were remodelling the NHS. In 1980 the concept was officially buried.[59] In future, the Government laid down, the maximum size for a DGH would normally be 600 beds, stressing at the same time the value of small, local hospitals. It was a decision which at one and the same time reflected the new philosophy of 'small is beautiful', rationalised the cuts in the capital investment programme and satisfied local political demands for accessible community hospitals.

The new emphasis on localism, and the reaction against expertise, was further reflected in a new permissiveness in planning. The document setting out the Conservative Government's priorities for the NHS published in 1981[60] marked a significant change from its predecessors published during the 1970s. The priorities themselves remained substantially unchanged, although there were some new themes such as the importance of co-operation between the NHS and the private sector. Like its predecessors the document – *Care in Action* – gave priority to the services for the elderly, mentally handicapped and other deprived groups. But if there was continuity in policy aims, there was a sharp break in the policy means. Unlike its predecessors, the 1981 document no longer expressed its priorities in terms of norms or financial targets: a reflection, in part, of the disillusionment with planning discussed in the previous section. Nor did it suggest how extra resources could be found for the priority services at a time of severe budgetary constraints, apart from the ritualistic invocation of the scope for greater efficiency. If the implementation of the priorities implied even tighter rationing in other service sectors, the responsibility was firmly delegated to the peripheral authorities. The Government, clearly, did not want to know. The only echo of the language of rational planning was the insistence on the importance of developing improved tools of analysis and information systems designed to assess the quality and efficiency of the services being provided.

In putting the stress on simplification and decentralisation as against central planning, the Conservative Government was largely acting within the new consensus that had developed in the second half of the 1970s. On one point, though, there was sharp disagreement: the constitution of the health authorities. While the 1974–79 Labour Government had, reluctantly, accepted the organisational framework created by Sir Keith Joseph, it had made one change: minor in its impact, but richly symbolic. The new authorities set up in 1974, the Labour Party argued, were undemocratic because appointive. So in 1975 the constitution of AHAs was changed to strengthen the representation of local authorities[61]: at least a third of all members were to be drawn from local government – on the principle, seemingly, that someone annointed with the holy oil of election for one purpose automatically became sanctified as an all-purpose democratic representative. At the same time, the Labour Government proposed that two further members in each AHA should be 'drawn from amongst those working in the NHS': so extending representation from doctors and nurses to other NHS workers. This proposal came to nothing because of disagreement among the trade unions, and between the trade unions and professional organisations, as to how these two worker representatives should be chosen.

On both counts, the 1982 model marked the rejection of Labour policies. The representation of local authorities on the DHAs has been reduced to a quarter of the total membership, and the idea of worker representation has been abandoned – although one member is appointed on the recommendation of the trade unions. However, the 'voice of the expert' remains represented: each DHA contains a consultant, a general practitioner and a nurse. If medical domination of the health authorities is numerically less visible than in the original NHS created by Bevan (see Ch. 2), medical representation continues to be institutionalised.

Like the original 1948 NHS and like the reorganised 1974 service, the 1982 NHS represents a compromise between competing ends and values. In order to achieve simplification, a price had to be paid: once again it proved impossible to reconcile the various desirable policy aims. The disappearance of AHAs meant the abandonment of shared boundaries between health and local authorities: if co-terminosity had not automatically led to greater collaboration, the new arrangement inevitably has introduced new administrative complexities into the search for co-operation. Similarly, the disappearance of AHAs signalled the abandonment of any hope of integrating the administration of general practice more closely into health service planning. Under the new system, Family Practitioner Committees have once again – like the original 1948 Executive Committees – become free-floating bodies. Both their boundaries and their finances are entirely independent of the DHAs. This not only represents an admission of defeat in the past – the fact that FPCs had remained stubbornly independent of AHAs; it also represents the acceptance of the fact that an attempt to integrate general practice into the NHS by abolishing the FPCs, as recommended by the Royal Commission, would carry excessive political costs by leading to a confrontation with general practitioners. Once again the medical profession had been able to veto change, not by opposing it explicitly but by constraining the concept of feasibility held by policy-makers.

Above all, the 1982 model leaves unresolved the basic dilemma of the relationship between the centre and the periphery: a dilemma which has haunted the NHS since its inception and which featured so prominently in the Cabinet debates of 1946 (see Ch. 1). Everybody paid verbal homage to the principle of decentralisation, but how was this going to be achieved in a nationally-financed service? 'I remain firmly convinced that the National Health Service is a noble concept but we can make it work a great deal better', Patrick Jenkin pronounced. 'First and foremost, I believe that we must see the NHS, not as a single national organisation, but as it is perceived by those who use it and those who work in it at the local level – as a series of local services run by local management, responsive to local needs and with a strong involvement from the local community.' The Secretary of State also recognised, however, the problem of squaring central accountability and the local autonomy: 'This is difficult in a service where virtually the entire finance comes from the centre – from the Exchequer. That is why in the longer term I think it right that we should examine whether it is not possible for more of the finance for the Health Service to be generated locally as they do in so many other countries.' So, inevitably, the attempt to solve organisational problems – to translate a new political ideology of disengagement into practice – led to the questioning of the financial basis of the NHS. The Conservative ideology in any case predisposed Ministers to search for alternatives to the inherited system of financing health care, with a strong bias (as we have seen) towards the private market. But this predisposition was further reinforced by the realisation that organisation and finance were the two sides of the same coin: political disengagement by central government could only follow financial disengagement.

Unsurprisingly, therefore, the Conservative Ministers embarked on a search for new methods of financing health services. But the only actual change introduced – apart from the familiar step of increasing the revenue from prescriptions and other charges – was to permit and encourage DHAs to engage in local fund-raising activities. Although denounced by the Labour Opposition as a return to the pre-1948 days, when voluntary hospitals had to generate funds by flag-days and bazaars, the impact of this change seems likely to be modest. In 1979–80, the total income from subscriptions, donations and legacies was £20 million. Even if this were to be doubled – or quadrupled – it would still represent only the small change of the NHS's total budget. However, the change provides further evidence of the shift in the Government's ideology. For it implies once again a shift from national uniformity as the overriding policy objective for the NHS to the acceptance of a greater degree of diversity, since the fund-raising capacity of DHAs is bound to vary. If hypocrisy is the tribute vice pays to virtue, symbolic action is the tribute political necessity pays to party ideology. Just as the Labour Ministers in 1974 felt compelled to take action on pay beds by the need to satisfy their political constituency, so the Conservative Ministers in 1979 were forced to make a show of their commitment to their party's new ideology. In both cases it proved more expedient to make changes which were ideologically resonant rather than financially or politically costly.

Overall, then, the real significance of the policy innovations and changes that have marked the start of the 1980s does not lie primarily in their direct effect on the structure, organisation and financing of the NHS. These have been marginal. It lies in the insights they provide into the changing nature of the health care policy arena. To summarise the arguments of this chapter, these were as follows. First, the arena has become more crowded with increasingly assertive actors. Second, the prevailing consensus has come under strain as political ideology has come to play a larger part: reflecting the wider political and economic environment. Third, the consensus itself has evolved: the faith of the creators of the NHS in rational planning, in giving free rein to the experts, has become eroded. Fourth, while in the post-war era of economic growth governments were anxious to centralise credit – to claim responsibility for the improvements made possible by increasing prosperity – the stress now is on diffusing blame for the inevitable shortcomings in an era of economic crisis: to decentralise responsibility is also to disclaim blame. Lastly, and perhaps most important, the combination of all these factors has been to put new issues on the NHS policy agenda: to set a question mark against assumptions which hitherto had seemingly been set in the concrete of a generally accepted conventional wisdom. If the consensus survives – changed, battered and motheaten – it can no longer be taken for granted.

REFERENCES

1. RUDOLF KLEIN, 'The Stalemate Society,' *Commentary*, Nov. 1973, pp. 42–7.
2. The analysis here draws on Samuel Beer, 'In search of a New Public Philosophy' in Anthony King (ed.), *The New American Political System*, American Enterprise Institute: Washington, D.C. 1978. Although Beer's analysis of the intellectual climate in the 1960s and 1970s is based on American experience, it is equally relevant to Britain.
3. MINISTRY OF HOUSING AND LOCAL GOVERNMENT, *People and Planning*, HMSO: London 1969.
4. F. W. S. CRAIG (ed.), *British General Election Manifestos, 1900–1974*, Macmillan: London 1975.
5. ANTHONY KING, 'Overload: Problems of Governing in the

1970s'; *Political Studies*, vol. XXIII, nos. 2–3, June–Sept. 1975, pp. 162–74.

6. ROBERT BACON and WALTER ELTIS, *Britain's Economic Problem: Too Few Producers*, Macmillan: London 1976.

7. CHANCELLOR OF THE EXCHEQUER, *Public Expenditure to 1979–80*, HMSO: London 1976, Cmnd. 6393.

8. SOCIAL SERVICES COMMITTEE Third Report, Session 1980–81, *Public Expenditure on the Social Services*, vol. 2, HMSO: London 1981, H.C. 324–11. Because of a change in the method of presenting figures in the Public Expenditure White Paper, the figure derived from this source is for England only.

9. BARBARA CASTLE, *The Castle Diaries, 1974–76*, Weidenfeld & Nicolson: London 1980. See App. 1 for expenditure figures.

10. EXPENDITURE COMMITTEE Ninth Report, Session 1976–77, *Spending on the Health and Personal Social Services*, HMSO: London 1977, H.C. 466; Social Services Committee Third Report, Session 1979–80, *The Government's White Papers on Public Expenditure: The Social Services*, HMSO: London 1980, H.C. 702.

11. DEPARTMENT OF HEALTH AND SOCIAL SECURITY, *The NHS Planning System*, HMSO: London 1976.

12. DEPARTMENT OF HEALTH AND SOCIAL SECURITY, *Priorities for Health and Personal Social Services in England*, HMSO: London 1976.

13. RUDOLF KLEIN, 'Ideology, Class and the National Health Service', *Journal of Health Politics, Policy and Law*, vol. 4, no. 3, Fall 1979, pp. 464–91.

14. NATIONAL BOARD FOR PRICES AND INCOMES Report no. 166, *The Pay and Conditions of Service of Ancillary Workers in the National Health Service*, HMSO: London 1971, Cmnd. 4644.

15. ROYAL COMMISSION on the National Health Service, *Report*, HMSO: London 1979, Cmnd. 7615.

16. RUDOLF KLEIN, 'Incomes: Vive La Différence', *British Medical Journal*, 10 July 1976, pp. 126–7. Strictly, the figures given in the text refer to the median quartile of people in each group.

17. REVIEW BODY ON DOCTORS' AND DENTISTS' REMUNERATION, *Sixth Report, 1976*, HMSO: London 1976, Cmnd. 6473.

18. REVIEW BODY ON DOCTORS' AND DENTISTS' REMUNERATION, *Seventh Report, 1977*, HMSO: London 1977, Cmnd. 6800.

19. REVIEW BODY ON DOCTORS' AND DENTISTS' REMUNERATION, *Eighth Report, 1978*, HMSO: London 1978, Cmnd. 7176.

20. REVIEW BODY ON DOCTORS' AND DENTISTS' REMUNERATION,

Tenth Report, 1980, HMSO: London 1980, Cmnd. 7903.
21. For a detailed narrative of this dispute see Susan Treloar, 'The Junior Hospital Doctors' Pay Dispute 1975–1976', *Journal of Social Policy,* vol. 10, no. 1, Jan. 1981, pp. 1–30.
22. BMJ, Report of proceedings of the Central Committee for Hospital Medical Services, *British Medical Journal,* 6 Dec. 1975, pp. 593–5.
23. Leading article, 'Industrial action by doctors', *British Medical Journal,* 6 Dec. 1975, p. 544.
24. SIR THEODORE FOX, 'Industrial Action, The National Health Service, and the Medical Profession', *The Lancet,* 23 Oct. 1976, pp. 892–5.
25. BMJ, 'Discussion document on ethical responsibilities of doctors practising in the National Health Service', *British Medical Journal,* 15 Jan. 1977, pp. 157–9.
26. BMJ, 'From the Council', *British Medical Journal,* 7 Oct. 1978, p. 1033.
27. BMJ, 'The Week', *British Medical Journal,* 3 June 1978, p. 1479.
28. RUDOLF KLEIN and JANET LEWIS, *The Politics of Consumer Representation,* Centre for Studies in Social Policy: London 1976.
29. KATHY SAYER, (ed.), *The King's Fund Directory of Organisations for Patients and Disabled People,* King Edward's Hospital Fund: London 1979.
30. The analysis draws on Rudolf Klein, 'Ideology, Class and the National Health Service', *op. cit.* Where no sources are given in the text, they can be found in this paper.
31. BARBARA CASTLE, *The Castle Diaries, op. cit.,* p. 131.
32. D. P. Choyce, Letter in the *British Medical Journal,* 21 August 1976, p. 479.
33. BARBARA CASTLE, *The Castle Diaries, op. cit.,* p. 568.
34. DEPARTMENT OF HEALTH AND SOCIAL SECURITY, *The Separation of Private Practice from National Health Service Hospitals: A Consultative Document,* DHSS: London 1975.
35. HEALTH SERVICES BOARD, *Annual Report, 1979,* HMSO: London 1980, H.C. 354.
36. For details of the contract, see Review Body on Doctors' and Dentists' Remuneration, *Ninth Report, 1979, op. cit.*
37. ROYAL COMMISSION ON THE NATIONAL HEALTH SERVICE, *Report, op. cit.*
38. ROYAL COMMISSION ON THE NATIONAL HEALTH SERVICE, Research Paper no. 5, *Patients' Attitudes to the Hospital Service,*

HMSO: London 1978; Research Paper no. 6, *Access to Primary Care*, HMSO: London 1978.

39. ROYAL COMMISSION ON THE NATIONAL HEALTH SERVICE, Research Paper no. 1, *The Working of the National Health Service* (Maurice Kogan *et al.*), HMSO: London 1978.

40. *Regional Chairmen's Enquiry into the Working of the DHSS in Relation to Regional Health Authorities*, DHSS: London 19 May 1976.

41. COMMITTEE OF PUBLIC ACCOUNTS, *Ninth Report, Session 1976–77*, HMSO: London 1977, H.C. 532.

42. EXPENDITURE COMMITTEE, Ninth Report, Session 1976–77, *Spending on the Health and Personal Social Services*, HMSO: London 1977, H.C. 466.

43. SOCIAL SERVICES COMMITTEE, Third Report, Session 1979–80, *The Government's White Papers on Public Expenditure: The Social Services*, HMSO: London 1980, H.C. 702.

44. SOCIAL SERVICES COMMITTEE, Third Report, Session 1980–81, *Public Expenditure on the Social Services*, HMSO: London 1981, H.C. 324.

45. DEPARTMENT OF HEALTH AND SOCIAL SECURITY, *The Way Forward*, HMSO: London 1977.

46. DAVID J. HUNTER, *Coping With Uncertainty*, Research Studies Press: Chichester 1980; R. G. S. Brown, *Reorganising the National Health Service*, Basil Blackwell/Martin Robertson: Oxford 1979; S. Hayward and A. Alaszewski, *Crisis in the Health Service*, Croom Helm: London 1980.

47. SOCIAL SERVICES COMMITTEE, Third Report, Session 1980–81, *op. cit.*, p. 104.

48. PETER D. FOX, 'Managing Health Resources: English Style' in Gordon McLachlan (ed.), *By Guess or By What? Information Without Design in the NHS*, Oxford U. P. 1978; Michael Butts, Doreen Irving and Christopher Whitt, *From Principles to Practice*, Nuffield Provincial Hospitals Trust: London 1981.

49. TIMOTHY BOOTH, 'Collaboration Between the Health and Social Services', pts 1 and 2, *Policy and Politics*, vol. 9, nos. 1 and 2, Jan. and April 1981, pp. 23–51 and 205–227.

50. CHANCELLOR OF THE EXCHEQUER, *The Government's Expenditure Plans, 1980–81 to 1983–84*, HMSO: London 1980, Cmnd. 7841.

51. ROYAL COMMISSION ON THE NATIONAL HEALTH SERVICE, *Research Paper no. 1, op. cit.*

52. COMMITTEE OF INQUIRY INTO NORMANSFIELD HOSPITAL, *Report*, HMSO: London 1978, Cmnd. 7357. See also Rudolf Klein, 'Normansfield: Vacuum of Management in the NHS', *British Medical Journal*, 23 Dec. 1978, pp. 1802–4.

53. JANE SMITH, 'Conflict Without Change: The Case of London's Health Services', *Political Quarterly*, vol. 52, no. 4, Oct. 1981.

54. N. KORMAN and H. SIMONS, 'Hospital Closures' in Royal Commission on the National Health Service, *Research Paper no. 1*, *op. cit.*

55. This analysis draws on Rudolf Klein, 'Health Services', Ch. 9 in P. M. Jackson (ed.), *Government Policy Initiatives 1979–80*, Royal Institute of Public Administration: London 1981. Where no sources are given in the text, they can be found in this paper.

56. DEPARTMENT OF HEALTH AND SOCIAL SECURITY, *Patients First*, HMSO: London 1979.

57. DEPARTMENT OF HEALTH AND SOCIAL SECURITY, *Health Service Development: Structure and Management*, Circular HC (80)8, July 1980.

58. *The Economist*, note on 'Health Services', 29 Aug. 1981, pp. 23–4.

59. DEPARTMENT OF HEALTH AND SOCIAL SECURITY, *Hospital Services: The Future Pattern of Provision in England*, DHSS: London May 1980.

60. DEPARTMENT OF HEALTH AND SOCIAL SECURITY, *Care in Action*, HMSO: London 1981. See also Rudolf Klein, 'The Strategy Behind the Jenkin Non-Strategy', *British Medical Journal*, 28 Mar. 1981, pp. 1089–91.

61. DEPARTMENT OF HEALTH AND SOCIAL SECURITY, *Democracy in the National Health Service*, HMSO: London 1974; Department of Health and Social Security, *Democracy in the National Health Service*, Circular HSC (IS)194, Sept. 1975.

Chapter five
TOWARDS A BALANCE SHEET

Has the National Health Service been a success? The question
has a seductive but deceptive simplicity, for it begs the much more
difficult and complex question of what criteria should be used in
assessing the success, or otherwise, of the NHS. Not only did the
creation of the NHS represent, as noted in Chapter 1, a compromise
between different political interests and values. But, as the subsequent analysis has demonstrated, those values themselves have come
under increasing challenge over the past decade as new interests have
asserted themselves. In a pluralistic society, the NHS inevitably
mirrors the tensions between competing concepts of the desirable
objectives of public policy. The politics of health care represent, to
a large extent, endeavours to impose rival definitions of what is
desirable. Any attempt to draw up a balance sheet therefore involves
disentangling the different criteria of success. For the record of the
NHS cannot be assessed in terms of a single currency of evaluation:
all that an attempt at evaluation can hope to achieve is to expose the
nature of the trade-offs between different values and the conclusions
that follow from different ways of looking at the achievements of the
NHS. This chapter will therefore draw together some of the themes
that have run through the analysis so far, since it is these which
illustrate the policy perceptions and policy dilemmas that have to be
taken into account in any exercise in evaluation.

The problems of assessing the achievements of the NHS are compounded, to reinforce a point stressed earlier, by the sheer scale,
complexity and heterogeneity of the services it provides. Some figures may help to convey a sense of what is involved in delivering
health services to a population of 50 million people.[1] The NHS owns
over 2,600 hospitals, with 450,000 beds. Every year these hospitals
deal with over 6 million in-patients and cope with 37 million out-
patient attendances. In turn, the hospital system breaks down into

36 different specialties, backed by a complex network of supporting facilities ranging from pathology to nuclear physics. Apart from 38,000 doctors and 415,000 nurses, the staff includes medical laboratory technicians, photographers and artists, physiotherapists, radiographers and remedial gymnasts, biochemists, physicists, psychologists, pharmacists, occupational therapists and orthoptists, as well as 113,000 administrative and clerical staff and 211,000 ancillary workers. In the primary care sector, 22,000 general practitioners issue some 300 million prescriptions a year, while health visitors and home nurses look after 7 million people in their own homes: and all this without even considering the dental, opthalmic and pharmaceutical services. The sheer diversity of the NHS – as reflected in this mixture of skills employed and services provided – complicates the task of assessment: in an organisation which copes with anything from deformed bunions to life-threatening heart attacks, no simple measure of success can be used to assess performance.

In one respect, however, the NHS can be confidently pronounced to be an unambiguous success. If the criterion of evaluation is political acceptability, then the NHS represents a major triumph in the post-war history of British policy initiatives. In a period of growing disenchantment with the policy and organisational experiments of successive governments, the NHS has remained largely immune from generic disillusionment, if not from specific criticism. It has proved remarkably effective in generating loyalty. Not only has satisfaction with the NHS been consistently high, to reiterate a theme which has run through this book, but it has also been relatively higher than that with other public services, such as education.[2] Whatever its strengths or weaknesses as an instrument for delivering health care, the NHS has thus been a successful instrument for delivering support to the political system.

The contribution of the NHS to the health of the political system (as distinct from the health of the people) goes deeper still, it may be argued. In the view of Titmuss,[3] for example, the very existence of the NHS – and its commitment to providing a universal and free service in response to need – affects the nature of the social consensus. It both expresses and reinforces a sense of individual altruism and collective responsibility. Consequently, it strengthens social cohesiveness and solidarity. From this perspective, the NHS represents an important collective good, even if it has not cured a single patient. It is a persuasive view but the evidence permits only an agnostic conclusion: in a sense, the claim is too large and general to permit it to be tested. All that we do know is that British society tends to be *less* altruistic and *more* individualistic than many other countries which do not have the same kind of national health service, for example when judged by their attitudes to the poor.[4] What we cannot know, of course, is whether such attitudes would be still more pronounced if it were not for the existence of the NHS. Perhaps the most that can be said is that the NHS may have a general social role, as a symbol of social reassurance, as well as specific functions, and that its popularity may reflect its success as much in the former as in the latter capacity.

Next, therefore, we turn to examining the record of the NHS in terms of various specific criteria of assessment. First, this chapter examines the performance of the NHS in the light of the policy aims of its creators, and what the performance tells us in turn about the realism and appropriateness of those aims. Second, it analyses the record of the NHS in the light of alternative ways of looking at the performance of health care systems.

UNIVERSALISING THE ADEQUATE

The first aim of the NHS, as spelled out by Bevan in 1948 (see Ch. 1), was achieved by the act of creation itself. The introduction of a free health service automatically meant that the ability to get treatment was divorced from the ability to pay. The financial barricades having been torn down, the way was open for achieving equity in the use of health services: of ensuring that the only criterion for treatment or care was need – that people with equal needs would be treated equally, irrespective of their income. In the outcome, however, it proved easier to introduce the policy means than to achieve the policy objectives: like other instruments of social engineering, such as comprehensive schools, the NHS continues to mirror the society in which it is anchored and to reflect the divisions within it.

The evidence about the NHS's record in achieving equity is both ambiguous and contentious. Nevertheless, two conclusions can be drawn with reasonable confidence. First, the NHS has very largely achieved equity in terms of access to services. There is no evidence of a social class bias in access to general practitioner services, and little evidence of such a bias in access to hospital services.[5] This conclusion would seem to hold even when account is taken of the fact that the poorest members of the population are also those most likely to have the worst health and thus the greatest need for medical care. Second, however, the NHS has been conspicuously less successful in achieving equity in terms of the quality of care provided once access to the system has been achieved. There is consistent evidence that the best-off members of the community get most out of the NHS in terms of the quality of service received. The evidence continues to support the view of Titmuss, put forward as long ago as 1968,[6] that: 'the higher income groups know how to make better use of the Service. They tend to receive more specialist attention; occupy more of the beds in better equipped and staffed hospitals; receive more elective surgery; have better maternity care, and are more likely to get psychiatric help and psychotherapy than low income groups – particularly the unskilled.'

This is not surprising. The architects of the NHS were remarkably innocent in their assumption that equity would be achieved merely by making the service free. Whether this was a necessary condition is debatable; that it was not a sufficient condition is certain. For even a free health service imposes costs on its users and requires an investment of resources by them. The currency of payment is no longer money but time; the resources required are no longer financial but social. If patients no longer have to pay to see their doctor, they do have to spend time queueing in the general practitioner's surgery or waiting for a hospital appointment or operation. If patients can no longer buy higher quality care in the NHS (leaving private practice out of account, for the moment), they require the ability to manipulate a bureaucratic environment in order to get the best out of the service.

The concept of non-financial costs and resources helps to explain both the NHS's success in bringing about equity in terms of access and its failure to bring about equity in terms of quality. It is the poorest members of the community, the old and the unemployed in particular, who are richest in time, and it is time-costs which are most important in determining access: if rationing is by queueing, then those with the most time are likely to get to the top. But it is the best-off members of the community who tend to have the resources of knowledge and the social skills required to make the best use of the health service once access has been gained: there is consistent cross-national evidence that, irrespective of the way in which health care is organised and financed in different countries, the best educated make the most intensive use of what is available.[7] So the limited success of the NHS in achieving equity, as between the various socio-economic groups in the country, should be seen not so much as a failure by the service as the almost inevitable reflection of inequalities in the distribution of articulacy, knowledge and social confidence.

Turning to Bevan's second aim, 'to provide the people of Great Britain, no matter where they may be, with the same level of service', the NHS can be pronounced only a qualified success: geographical equity, too, still remains to be fully achieved. At the start of the NHS's history the movement towards equity in the geographical distribution of revenue and capital funds was, as we have seen, inhibited by the overriding urgency of patching up the threadbare fabric inherited by the NHS. At the end of our period, the movement was inhibited by financial stringency, organisational rigidity and the strength of the constituencies for the *status quo*. The NHS therefore continues to be marked by considerable, if lessening, variations in the availability of services as well as diversity in the way resources are used. The variations in the resources inherited by the Area Health Authorities when they were set up in 1974, noted earlier, had only marginally diminished by the end of the decade. Taking county areas, Wiltshire's budget represented an income of £156 per head of population, while that of Suffolk was only £110. Taking urban areas, at one extreme we find inner-London AHAs like Kensington and Chelsea with an income of £317 and Camden and Islington with an income of £292. At the other extreme, there is Sandwell with an income of £88 and North Tyneside with an income of £92.[8] These figures exaggerate the differences in the services available to the populations concerned. The high spenders tend to be authorities with a heavy concentration of teaching hospitals which import patients outside their own boundaries; the low spenders tend to export many of their patients to neighbouring, better-equipped authorities. But, making every allowance for such distortions, the evidence confirms the persistence of inequalities in the distribution of resources.

Inequalities in the distribution of resources are compounded by differences in local policies and clinical practices. For example, while the relatively under-provided Trent region provides hospital in-patient treatment for appendicitis at a rate of 12.7 cases per 10,000 population, the equivalent figure for the relatively over-provided North-East Thames region is 16.0; while the West Midlands region, towards the bottom end of the resource league, provides hospital in-patient treatment for varicose veins at the rate of 4.9 cases per 10,000 population, the equivalent figure for the South-East Thames region, nearer the top of the resource league, is 9.7.[9] To an extent, the kind of treatment people get still depends on where they live. Difference does not, however, necessarily mean inequity. The figures of differences in the numbers of particular operations carried out, quoted above, could be supplemented by figures showing differences also in the waiting times, in the availability of medical staff and the lengths of stay in hospital. Once again, however, the principle of infinite diversity has to be invoked. If one hospital or district chooses to provide in-patient treatment for varicose veins, another may treat them on a day care basis; if one doctor automatically whips all his patients with a heart attack into hospital, another may treat them in their own homes. In short, the experience of the NHS would seem to suggest that its architects seriously underestimated the difficulties – as much conceptual as organisational or financial – of achieving geographical equity in the strict sense of ensuring equal access to equal levels of service for people in equal need. Given the fact that there is much scope for substituting different kinds of service, given the lack of medical consensus about what is an appropriate package of care for any specific condition and given that definitions of need vary over time and with the perceptions of individual clinicians, it is not surprising that the NHS has found this philosopher's stone somewhat elusive.

In any case, if the NHS's record in moving towards geographical equity is disappointing when measured against the expectations of its architects, it is a striking success story when measured against the achievements of most other countries. The problem of maldistribution is international. In so far as it is possible to draw any conclusions from the available data, the variations in Britain appear to be less conspicuous than in most other developed countries: even in Russia, where there is a totally planned economy, large-scale geographical variations persist.[10] In the case of the NHS, it can at least be said that there is nothing wrong with the policy instruments for promoting progress towards the achievement of geographical equity which could not be cured by a faster economic growth rate: by factors outside the control of the health care policy-makers.

One exception must, however, be made to this assertion. In the case of general practice in Britain geographical variations in the distribution of doctors have persisted throughout the history of the NHS.[11] Despite the existence of a machinery for limiting the entry of new GPs into over-doctored parts of the country, despite the existence of financial incentives designed to encourage new GPs to settle in the under-doctored parts of the country, the variations have not been eliminated – though they have grown less gross over time. Here the constraint on achieving a better distribution is not lack of resources but professional attitudes. Once again, it is important to stress that this is an international problem whose causes should therefore not be sought in weaknesses inherent in the NHS or in attitudes specific to the British medical profession: doctors everywhere (including Russia) appear to be reluctant to move to those parts of the country which they consider to be less attractive or less remunerative. If money is mobile, medical manpower is not necessarily so.

The inability to eliminate variations within the NHS provides an illuminating footnote to the 1946 Cabinet debate between Bevan and Morrison (see Ch. 1). Bevan's main argument, it will be remembered, was that a national service was required if inequalities between the poor and rich parts of the country were not to be perpetuated: local government control, he maintained, was incompatible with this objective. Yet ironically central government has, in the outcome, been more successful in reducing the variations in the distribution of resources in at least some local authority services, such as education, than in the NHS.[12] For example, the distribution of teachers is more even than that of general practitioners. This suggests that there are factors specific to the health care policy arena, overriding the particular organisational form of the service, which create special difficulties in the way of achieving geographical equity.

First, the comparison between the NHS and education would seem to reinforce the conclusion that there are conceptual problems specific to health care which compound the difficulty of successfully implementing resource allocation policies. In the case of education, there is no difficulty in defining the client population: the law automatically determines the number of children who have to be schooled. Need thus defines itself, and permits a simple allocative principle to be used: the teacher – pupil ratio. The actual ratio chosen may, to an extent, be arbitrary: but conceptual simplicity simplifies the task of policy implementation in the case of education, just as conceptual complexity compounds the problems in the case of health.

Second, the comparison between the NHS and education would seem to indicate a crucial difference in the power of the professionals in the two services. In the case of the NHS, the medical profession has succeeded in exercising tight control over the production of doctors. For most of the history of the NHS, demand for medical manpower has exceeded the supply of home-trained doctors[13]: the result both of professional pressures and of miscalculations about the number of doctors likely to be needed. The shortfall has been met by drawing in doctors from overseas, who tend to find jobs in the least popular specialties and the least popular parts of the country. In the case of education, however, the story is different: there has been an over-production of home-trained teachers, largely reflecting assumptions about the future size of the school population which subsequently turned out to be wrong. One reason for the better distribution of teachers may therefore be that policy has been able to exploit the 'over-spilling bath' principle: if there is an excess of teachers, the surplus will almost certainly seep into the least attractive parts of the country. In contrast, the medical profession's control over entry – its insistence on matching the production of doctors to the availability of jobs – has until the 1980s at least ensured that distributional policies have to cope with overall shortages rather than surpluses, so compounding the difficulties of achieving Bevan's aim of ensuring the 'same level of service' throughout the country.

Of course, Bevan had a further, still more ambitious aim. This was to 'universalise the best'. In retrospect, this can be seen to be an aim incapable of fulfilment, because it was (and remains) totally incompatible with the financial basis of the NHS. Universalising the best assumes unlimited resources: an open cheque on the national purse. In practice, as we have seen, the NHS has become an instrument for rationing scarce resources. Its achievement lies not in universalising the best – a flamboyant piece of political rhetoric devoid of real meaning – but in universalising the adequate. If the NHS does not represent a total triumph for those who saw the new institution as a monument to Socialism, it does represent a success for those who saw it as an opportunity to rationalise the delivery of health care. If there are still differences in the distribution of resources, at least there is an assured minimum of service provision: specialist care is assured to everyone everywhere. 'Acute hospital services are generally excellent', the Royal Commission concluded.[14] If there are still glaring inadequacies in certain services within the NHS, the conspicuous over-consumption of medical technology has been successfully controlled. If there are still queues for some operations, if there is still an unsatisfied demand for treatment, at least everyone who is acutely ill can be assured of immediate attention. Finally, if universalising adequacy may seem a somewhat modest achievement in terms of the expectations held in 1948, it represents a very considerable achievement when Britain's health care system is compared to that of other countries – where the search for adequate minimum standards of health care provision still continues.[15]

PRODUCERS v. CONSUMERS: WHO DECIDES WHAT IS BEST?

So far the achievements of the NHS have been analysed exclusively through the perceptual lenses of its architects. But the creation of the NHS reflected, as argued in Chapter 1, a very specific way of looking at the problem of designing a health care system, embodying a particular set of values. It represented the rejection of the market principle in favour of a collectivist solution. Implicit in this were two sets of assumptions. First was the assumption that there is a collective interest in the provision of health care, over and above the self-interest of individual members of society. Second, there was the assumption that health care is different in as much as the consumer does not know best: a market solution was rejected precisely because, it was argued, buying health care was not like buying a car, refrigerator or having one's boiler repaired. The consumer does not have adequate information to make sensible judgements, and a mistake once made cannot be put right by trading in the defective or unsatisfactory product for another (that is, many forms of medical intervention may well be irreversible). So, in short, the presumption must be that it is the producer – not the consumer – who knows best what requires to be done.

The logic of this argument for a collectivist solution is, however, also the logic of justification for a paternalistic approach to the provision of health care. If the language of demands is that of the market, the language of needs is that of paternalism. If the market assumes consumer sovereignty, paternalism assumes producer sovereignty. Moreover, while the market has a pluralistic bias, paternalism has a monistic bias. If there is such a thing as an ideal health policy – for example, equity in meeting expert-defined need – then the normal processes of pluralistic bargaining in the political market place would seem to be irrelevant. Indeed, accepting the case for paternalism would seem to imply accepting also the case for the private government of public health by those who know best. So it is perhaps not surprising that, as we have seen, the arena of health care policy was characterised – at least until the 1970s – by the dominance of the paternalist rationalisers in what was largely a self-contained, introspective world. However, as also noted, the dominance of the paternalist rationalisers – of the technocratic planners – has come under increasing challenge as the health care policy arena opened up. In turn, this would suggest a rather different perspective on evaluation from that used in the previous section: a perspective which involves asking whether the NHS has succeeded in meeting demands rather than needs.

In trying to answer this question, there is an obvious problem. To what extent does it make sense to use the language of the market in the context of health care? If there is an inevitable imbalance in the information available to the consumers and producers of health care, as there undoubtedly is, does it not then follow that the demands of the former will be shaped by the latter? The experience of the NHS would seem to support this view: in a sense, the NHS is a very successful machine for shaping – and limiting – demand. The only point where the consumer makes a demand on the NHS is when he or she visits the general practitioner: thereafter, decisions about the kind and level of treatment offered are made by the professional providers. Significantly, there has actually been a fall in the average annual number of general practitioner consultations made by the population of Britain over the history of the NHS[16]: the increase in activity has been confined to the hospital sector, reflecting demands from professionals, not consumers. Nor is this surprising. The incentive to the general practitioner in the NHS is to minimise his or her work: given that earnings are not related to the services performed, the general practitioner has an incentive to maximise his or her leisure rather than to maximise medical activity – either by damping patient expectations or by exporting problem cases into the hospital sector.

However, there is at least some independent evidence about the demand for health care, This comes from the private sector. For the private market in health care, by its very existence, indicates the scale and nature of the demands which are not satisfied by the NHS. It can thus be used, if only in a very rough and ready way, to assess the shortcomings of the NHS as perceived by those consumers who can afford to opt out of the national system. For example, as we saw in Chapter 3, the growth of abortion facilities in the private sector reflected the failure of the NHS to meet the demand generated by a change in legislation. The information available about the private market's activities is limited and patchy; however, it permits at least some tentative conclusions. First, the scale of private medical practice in Britain is small. Estimates vary, but there is agreement that total spending on private medical care (whether in NHS hospitals or in private surgeries and hospitals) accounts for between three and five per cent of the NHS's budget. Second, private practice appears to be on the increase: in part, this is the perverse policy outcome of the Labour Government's decision to phase out pay beds from NHS hospitals, which gave private entrepreneurs an incentive to develop new facilities. Between 1955 and 1980 the number of persons covered by insurance schemes which pay the cost of private medical treatment rose from 585,000 to 3,577,000: the increase between 1976 and 1980 being over 1,300,000.[17] These figures are not easy to interpret. This trend reflects the growth of company schemes which provide medical insurance as a fringe benefit for their (mainly) white-collar employees. In contrast, the number of individuals taking out their own insurance policies has tended to remain static. It is therefore difficult to distinguish between the effect of changes in company policies and changes in individual preferences as between the private and public sectors of health care.

However, the nature of the demands being met by the private sector is reasonably clear. Overwhelmingly, though not exclusively, the private market provides medical care for people of working age, suffering from relatively minor conditions, who want to be treated by their own consultant in a room of their own at a time of their own choice.[18] In other words, private patients are buying priority, privacy and treatment tailored to their own convenience rather than to that of the organisation providing the service. Conversely, the private sector tends to deal not with life-threatening acute conditions, requiring the technological resources usually only found in NHS hospitals, but with those conditions which cause disability or discomfort. Nor, on the whole, does it deal with the chronic degenerative diseases of old age: most insurance policies do not provide coverage for these.

All this would seem to suggest that the NHS is failing to meet consumer demands in a number of respects. It indicates that the NHS is giving less priority than many of its consumers would like to deal with discomfort-causing or work-disabling conditions: for example, the median waiting time for having a hernia repaired in the NHS is over 10 weeks, while that for having a cataract treated is 14 weeks. Inevitably the NHS gives less weight to the economic costs of delay, such as loss of earnings, than the individuals concerned. The organisational imperative is, after all, to give priority to medically-defined need, not to maintaining a healthy labour force: at any one time almost two-thirds of all the beds in acute hospitals are occupied by men and women over 60 (a reminder also that the NHS is an important instrument for re-distributing resources from the working to the non-working population).

Equally, the demand for private care indicates that the NHS is giving less priority than many of its consumers would like to providing them with a room of their own and individually-tailored treatment. The large ward remains the norm in the NHS, although there is a small number of amenity beds which offer privacy. Once again the explanation would seem to lie in organisational imperatives: to minimise the work falling on producers while maximising the output of patients. In the case of the large ward, for instance, it is argued that this makes the most efficient use of nurses. Given overall resource scarcity in the NHS, one rationing strategy is clearly to limit the time given to any one patient, to substitute as far as possible standard routines for treatment specifically adapted to the individual patient. In part, then, the demand for private care can be seen as a protest against such organisational routines.

There is, additionally, evidence from within the NHS which supports this interpretation. A survey of patients conducted on behalf of the Royal Commission,[19] while confirming overall satisfaction with the NHS, also showed considerable discontent with producer-imposed routines. Lack of privacy was a frequent complaint, though few patients actually wanted a room of their own. Two-fifths of those interviewed grumbled about being woken too early, not surprisingly since the majority of patients are woken up before 6.30 a.m. (with not a few being woken up at 5.30 a.m. so as to allow the night nurses to smarten up the patients before handing over to the day staff). Many, too, were dissatisfied with both the quality and the quantity of the information given to them by doctors and others about their progress. A third felt that they had been treated as 'just another case', not as individuals. Moreover, in the 1980s, as in the 1950s (see Ch. 2), organisational routines continue to provide obstacles in the way of making it easier for parents to visit, and stay with, their children in hospital: although practice has become far more liberal, it continues to lag behind the guidelines laid down by the DHSS[20]. While central government may exhort, it is the service professionals at the periphery who decide.

The private sector can thus be seen as an opportunity for consumers to voice those demands which are frustrated in the NHS; moreover, its activities can also be seen as a way of measuring the shortcomings of the NHS. But, it may be argued, the private sector contributes towards shortcomings by its very existence. It encourages NHS producers to ignore consumer demands. If the most articulate and demanding patients exit into the private sector, then the NHS is rid of its most troublesome customers. Conversely, if the most articulate and demanding patients were denied the exit option, they would be forced to use voice: to engage in the politics of protest.[21] The private sector, it can thus be argued, helps to sustain producer dominance in the NHS and to limit the demands for improvements. From this perspective, the perpetuation of a private market for health care constrains the development of a political market within the NHS.

This may, however, be an over-simple view. The ability to exercise voice – to protest – may, in fact, depend on the ability to exit from the NHS, as one political scientist has pointed out on the basis of his own experience as a dissatisfied patient.[22] If patients are often reluctant to complain or protest, it may be for fear of retaliation from the staff. If the NHS were to have a total monopoly of health care, the risk of retaliation would be compounded, and with it the inhibitions on using voice. Moreover, if we take the private sector seriously as an indicator of where the NHS is failing to satisfy demands, it is clear that increasing its responsiveness to consumer preferences would lead to a reversal of the present policies designed to favour the most deprived client group. What the most articulate and demanding consumers want, it would appear, is more facilities for elective surgery and better conditions in acute hospitals. But this could only be achieved, within the constraints of the NHS budget, at the expense of services for the old, the mentally handicapped and so on: those services where the consumers are least articulate and least demanding. In short, adopting a market perspective, and using consumer demand as the criterion of evaluation, would lead to the conclusion that the NHS has failed to give adequate priority to the acute services. This is just the reverse of the conventional wisdom which holds that the real failure of the NHS lies in investing too much in the acute services at the expense of those for the deprived groups – a view held, as we have seen, by a succession of both Conservative and Labour Ministers.

Two conclusions would seem to follow from this discussion of what the role of the private sector tells us about the performance of the NHS. The first is that the relationship between the two sectors is symbiotic. Each needs the other. For the NHS, the private sector provides an invaluable safety value. If the public sector is to go on rationing resources according to non-market criteria of need, then inevitably some demands will be frustrated: better that such demands be syphoned off into the market sector than that they should throw grit into the organisational machinery of the NHS. For the private sector, equally, the NHS is essential. If the NHS did not cope with the burden of providing medical care for the very ill, the very old and the very handicapped – those groups with the least market power – the private sector would have to accept responsibilities for which it is not equipped and which might not be very profitable either. Perhaps this helps to explain why, despite the ideological fury aroused by the issue of private practice, the relationship between the public and the private sectors of health has changed so remarkably little during the history of the NHS: the reality of mutual exploitation to mutual advantage has, so far at least, proved stronger than political rhetoric.

The second conclusion is that there is an inbuilt tension in the NHS. On the one hand, the real justification of the NHS lies precisely in the fact that it does not respond readily to consumer demands: that it is a device for compelling collective altruism in favour of the least powerful and most vulnerable. On the other hand, it is under increasing pressure to become more responsive. However, the logic of adopting consumer preferences as the guiding principle for the organisation of health care is to abolish the NHS and to replace it by a market-based system. In such a system the consumer (always assuming, heroically, that he or she has the necessary resources of finance and know-how) would be sovereign: producers would be forced to respond to market signals.[23] It would be consumer decisions, not political decisions about budgets and priorities, which would determine how much was spent, and on what.

Analytically, therefore, the languages of need and demand are incompatible: they reflect different values and point to different policy solutions. But politically, the history of the NHS shows a continuing attempt to blend them into a neutral policy Esperanto. In a sense the NHS consensus has been based on the assumption that the paternalism and consumerism can be combined: that there is no need to choose. The Labour Party has been reluctant to follow the logic of the language of need into embracing overt paternalism; the Conservative Party has been reluctant to follow the logic of the language of demand into embracing a market model of health care. In contrast to private practice, the very real ideological divide has been left implicit, blurred and fudged. It may be that the increasing fragility of the consensus, noted in the previous chapter, reflects the increasing instability of this compromise. It is indeed, tempting to argue that the dilemma can be resolved, and the historic compromise saved, by invoking the political market: by substituting political participation for consumer demands. If a solution based on consumer demand in the market place is rejected – on the grounds that this would simply reinforce the effects of inequalities in resources, both financial and social – a solution based on citizen demand expressed in the political market would seem to offer a viable alternative. Such a solution would appear to have the attraction of combining national decisions about priorities, in the light of defined need, with responsiveness to citizen preferences as expressed through participation in the political market.

This is, however, to change the vocabulary of discussion, not to resolve the underlying policy dilemma. The imbalances of the political market, to recapitulate the arguments advanced in previous chapters, are very similar to the imbalances in the economic market. Not only is there an imbalance between the concentrated interest group of health service producers and the diffuse and heterogeneous interest group of health service users,[24] but within the health service user group, the distinctions made in the context of the economic market carry over into the political market. It is precisely those who exit into the private sector – the most demanding and the most articulate citizens – who would be most capable of exercising voice in the political market. So we are back to the conclusion that encouraging political demands would run counter to policies designed to favour the most vulnerable: those with the least political resources. The inequalities in voice may, as we have seen, be attenuated by rigging the political market; by inventing institutions like Community Health Councils or encouraging pressure groups acting on behalf of the deprived. It is difficult, however, to see how they could be eliminated. Inescapably, the NHS has to live with the tensions between paternalism and participation, centralism and localism: tensions which do not represent a flaw in its achievements but are the inevitable consequences of trying to incorporate a number of competing policy aims in the same organisational structure.

MAKING THE EXPERTS ACCOUNTABLE

If the NHS remains quintessentially a service which meets expert-defined need rather than consumer-generated demands, this inevitably raises a further issue: an issue which, in retrospect, was curiously neglected in the discussions leading up to the creation of the service. To whom are the experts accountable? No attempt to assess the performance of the NHS in the 1980s can avoid trying to answer this question. The growing revolt against technical expertise, identified in the previous chapter, means that the NHS's claims to authority are no longer unchallenged. To the extent that the definition of need is problematic – reflecting changing professional perceptions and practices, rather than immutable scientific principles – so it is a political act in the widest sense: in the NHS, it is tempting to say with only a little exaggeration, he who defines need also has power.

At this point in the argument, it is crucial to distinguish sharply between two sets of experts. First, there are the *bureaucratic experts*: civil servants and the NHS administrators. Second, there are *professional experts*: doctors and other service providers. The paradox of the NHS is, to sum up the evidence of the previous chapters, that while it is the professional expert who decides which patient gets what in the way of treatment, the machinery of accountability is designed only to make the bureaucratic expert answerable for what he or she does. While the bureaucratic experts may be charged with increasing efficiency, the professional experts are intent to safeguard their autonomy: the values of bureaucratic rationalism and professional mystique are in conflict. In terms of accountability there is therefore a disjunction between the formal machinery and actual responsibility for making the decisions that matter most to the individual patient.

In theory, as we have seen, the NHS's system of administrative and financial accountability is clear and comprehensive. The Secretary of State is accountable to Parliament for every administrative decision, every penny spent, in the NHS. In turn all the health authorities – whether at regional or at district level – are accountable to the Secretary of State. Finally, to complete the circle of accountability, the bureaucratic experts are answerable to their various authorities. It is precisely this principle, of course, which has been at the root of the continuing debate since 1948 about the relationship between centre and periphery: the rhetoric of decentralisation inevitably comes into collision with the fact of accountability. In practice, as we have also seen, theory is often betrayed by practice. The relationship between the Secretary of State and his bureaucratic experts, the civil servants, may be strictly hierarchical in theory. But in reality, as both the Crossman and the Castle diaries make clear, he is also dependent on them. Given the sheer complexity and heterogeneity of the NHS, a Secretary of State cannot hope to know everything that goes on in his department. Parliamentary questions, or public scandals, may activate the machinery of accountability: but the process, at best, provides only a fitful, erratic searchlight lighting different parts of the NHS while leaving the rest of the landscape in the dark. It is, in short, a system of accountability designed more to investigate mistakes than to ensure that the positive aims of policy are being met: once again, we are back to the underlying problem posed by the lack of indicators of performance and the ambiguity of the available information.

Precisely the same point applies in the case of the regional and district authorities. The case of Normansfield, cited in the previous chapter, is only one example of the failure of health authority members to act as effective links in the chain of accountability. Nor is this surprising. If it is difficult for a full-time Secretary of State to exercise control, the problem is compounded in the case of part-time authority members. If there is an imbalance in the information available to consumers and producers, there is also an imbalance as between the controllers and the controlled. The principle of infinite diversity offers an open licence to diverge from national guidelines or national policies: to subvert accountability seen as responsibility for the implementation of specific policies. To over-simplify only a little, the bureaucratic experts of the NHS are accountable in terms of process – the propriety and equity with which policies are administered – not in terms of outcome. This may be inevitable given the fact that the bureaucratic experts have no authority over the professional experts. If the administrative hierarchy of the NHS is responsible for the allocation of resources (and accordingly accountable to Parliament), it is the professional providers who are responsible for the use of those resources: the dilemma noted already in Chapter 2. So to whom are the professional experts accountable? In trying to answer this question, we shall concentrate on the medical profession, given its crucial role and given the fact that other aspiring or would-be professions in the health care policy arena, such as nurses, tend to take doctors as their model.

Again, the theory of medical accountability is clear. Implicit in it is the notion of a collective contract between the profession and the public. In return for control of entry, effective monopoly rights over the exercise of its skills and immunity from lay scrutiny, the profession agrees to regulate itself: as members of a profession, doctors are accountable to their peers. The point was clearly put by the Merrison Committee, which reported on the regulation of the medical profession in 1975: 'An instructive way of looking at regulation is to see it as a contract between public and profession, by which the public go to the profession for medical treatment because the profession has made sure that it will provide satisfactory treatment.'[25] The main instrument of regulation is the General Medical Council, the subject of the Merrison inquiry: a body composed of members elected by the medical profession and nominated by educational institutions, with a small dash of nominated lay members. Its functions are twofold. First, it exists to make sure that those admitted to the medical register are competent. Second, it is charged with removing from the register 'those practitioners unfit to practice', to quote the Merrison report. Its role, in this latter capacity, is to deal with those doctors 'whose condition or conduct represents a general public risk'.

Does the official machinery of accountability actually ensure that the public can rely on getting 'satisfactory treatment' from members of the medical profession? The answer is, almost certainly, no. Once a doctor has graduated onto the medical register, the GMC's role is essentially negative. It reacts to complaints, whether from members of the public or from professional colleagues of the doctor concerned. Its role is to drum convicted sinners out of the profession, not to ensure continued professional virtue. The point is well illustrated by looking at the cases considered by the GMC in one year, 1980.[26] Altogether 113 cases were considered. The allegations were all about the doctors' personal conduct: 45 of them involved the abuse of alcohol and drugs, while a further 23 involved charges such as dishonesty, violence and indecency. In short, the GMC tends to deal with incompetence reflected in, and perhaps caused by, personal failings. Its machinery is not designed to deal with the doctor who is neither psychiatrically ill nor dishonest, who does not touch drink or drugs, who does not sleep with his patients or break the law, but has simply lost interest in his profession: who is a good and sane citizen but a poor doctor. If a doctor prefers to spend his time on the golf course rather than reading medical journals, that is of no concern to the GMC.

Equally limited in scope, and somewhat different in its intent, is the quite separate mechanism for holding general practitioners accountable. The system for investigating complaints against general practitioners was originally introduced in 1913 and was taken over virtually unchanged when the Family Practitioner Committees replaced Executive Councils in 1974.[27] The complaints are heard by a panel composed half of doctors and half of laymen. The whole procedure revolves around a very limited concept of accountability: its purpose is to hold general practitioners accountable for fulfilling the terms of their contract with the FPC (a similar procedure is available for the other professionals, for dentists, pharmacists and opticians, who are in a contractual relationship with the FPC.) The question being asked is whether the doctor has carried out the duties for which he is being paid, not whether he is a competent practitioner. Thus the complaints typically tend to involve such issues as the refusal of the doctor to visit his patients at home, the failure to issue medical certificates or to refer patients to hospital and inadequate or incorrect treatment. The last category touches, of course, on competence. But once again, the crucial point is that the role of FPCs is exclusively reactive. FPCs have neither the power nor the responsibility to hold doctors accountable for the way in which they practice.

In the case of the hospital service, the Health Service Commissioner – whose office was created in 1974 to provide a statutory back-up to the existing, non-statutory machinery for dealing with complaints in the NHS – is explicitly barred from considering complaints involving clinical discretion. Essentially his remit is to consider complaints involving the administration of health services: thus he may criticise a doctor for being slow to turn out of bed in response to an emergency, or being surly in manner, but not for actions 'taken solely in the exercise of clinical judgement'. About a fifth of the 600 or so complaints received by the Health Service Commissioner every year are rejected on the grounds that they involve questions of clinical judgement and are thus outside his jurisdiction.[28] It is a limitation whose introduction represented a victory for the medical profession's insistence that only doctors can judge the performance of other doctors, and which has been fiercely defended since. In 1977 a Parliamentary Committee recommended that the Health Service Commissioner's brief should be extended to cover cases involving clinical judgements, with an infusion of medical expertise into the investigative process.[29] But this recommendation stubbed its toe against the medical profession's stonewalling opposition to any hint of lay participation in medical accountability. Not until 1981 was a compromise cobbled up, which provided for the introduction of a machinery for dealing with complaints about the quality of treatment: a machinery which, however, was entirely controlled by the medical profession itself. Any system of accountability based on responding to complaints is, at best, incomplete: once again, it represents accountability for mistakes made, not accountability for the quality of the services delivered. But the history of the wrangle over the complaints machinery is instructive on two counts. It demonstrates the continuing veto-power of the medical profession on issues central to it. Equally, it shows the medical profession responding to the changes in the health care policy arena: forced to take pre-emptive action in order to fend off what might be more threatening and insistent demands.

The profession's sensitivity to the potential threats posed both by the bureaucratic expert's drive to secure more efficiency and by the assertive consumerism that was emerging in the 1970s is also reflected in its growing interest in the concept of medical audit or peer group review[30]: the idea that doctors should systematically review each other's performance. This was by no means an entirely novel concept. Indeed in the United States peer group review had long been standard practice. Even in Britain a systematic review of all deaths in the maternity services had already been launched in the 1950s: an exercise designed to identify avoidable causes of mortality. But the hope, expressed by the DHSS's Chief Medical Officer, Sir George Godber, in 1972 that 'other comparable exercises will become part of the Health Service in future',[31] had not been realised by the end of the decade. The new-found enthusiasm for collective self-assessment can therefore be seen – in part at least – as the profession's answer to the demand for a greater accountability.

The medical profession's enthusiasm was qualified, however. Its reservations emerge clearly from the report of a committee set up to 'review the present methods of ensuring the maintenance of standards of continuing competence to practice and of the clinical care of patients'.[32] This argued that the point of assessment should be to educate the doctor not to control him: 'We would stress that the purpose of both peer group and self assessment for practising doctors should be educational, and that any implication that sanctions may be deployed against those who appear to do less well than their colleagues would be damaging to such activities.' Similarly all attempts to devise or impose norms of efficient practice should be resisted: 'Studies have shown that the most significant factor in how hospital beds are used is the standard practice of the consultant in charge, yet little is known about the practice of one consultant compared with that of others, apart from simple quantitative variations in their use of such resources as hospital beds. There is insufficient evidence from studies of such variations to warrant a demand for conformity.'

Such an approach, while it may well help to improve standards of practice, leaves two critical problems untouched. First, it does nothing to deal with those doctors who do not want to take part in any assessment procedures: it leaves open the possibility that the most competent doctors (and most prestigious institutions) will use the mirror of peer review, while the least competent doctors (and least prestigious institutions) will avert their gaze from their own performance. In short, the good may become better, while the bad remains untouched. Second, the approach leaves unanswered the question of what criteria should be used in assessing the performance of doctors. Should the only criteria used be those of technical excellence? Or should they also take into account the use of resources?

In short, is the doctor responsible only for the quality of the medical care he gives to the patient in front of him, or does he also have responsibilities to those in the queue for resources? If his only responsibility is to maximise quality for the individual patient, then only exclusively technical criteria are relevant in any review exercise. If the aim is to maximise the health of any given population, then a different set of criteria may have to be invoked: criteria which involve social, economic and moral judgements, not just medical expertise. At the heart of the debate about accountability in health care there is, therefore, ambiguity as to what its purpose should be: whether it is accountability for individual acts or for collective, overall performance.

In concluding this discussion of the dilemmas of accountability in the NHS, it is important to stress that they are in no sense unique to the health service. What clinical discretion is for doctors, the secret garden of the curriculum is for teachers. Just as the medical profession resists any attempt to make it accountable for what doctors actually do, so teachers have fought political influence on the content, as distinct from the organisation and financing, of education. Neither, in turn, is the difficulty of introducing effective systems of accountability attributable to the monopoly power of professions in general or the special political strength of the medical profession. The police force offers a striking demonstration of how the power of non-professional service providers can be used to frustrate attempts to make them accountable: even consultants might hesitate before asserting their claim to autonomy in as ruthless a fashion as Chief Constables. In this respect, as in others, the NHS can therefore most usefully be seen as illuminating some general issues of political control in complex organisations where it is difficult to define aims, or to decide on the currency of accountability, and where the reality of effective power does not obediently follow constitutional doctrine.

WHAT USE IS THE NHS, ANYWAY?

During its lifespan the NHS's budget has, in real terms, almost tripled. The proportion of a growing national income devoted to the NHS has risen from under 4 per cent to 5.6 per cent. The NHS employs far more people and treats far more patients than when it was set up. The range and sophistication of the services offered has increased out of all recognition. Viewed from the organisation's own perspectives, this is undoubtedly a success story. If we accept the organisational imperative of maximising the opportunities for professional service providers, if the NHS is seen as a machine for discovering both new needs and new ways of meeting them, then the only flaw in its achievement is the fact that it has not got more resources: that its activities are constrained by a shortage of funds.

Increasingly, however, the organisational imperatives of the NHS have come under attack: new perspectives offer new criteria of assessment. The political reaction against the values of expertise, technology and bureaucracy, discussed in the previous chapter, reflected also an intellectual challenge to the values of professionalism as embodied in the NHS. No longer were the activities of the NHS seen as self-justifying. No longer was the authority of the medical profession in defining need accepted without question. On the contrary, the new criticism – a coalition of social scientists, philosophic anarchists and medical historians[33] – questioned the very assumptions on which the NHS was built. Medical intervention, it was argued, was a frequently misguided and sometimes damaging attempt to impose technical solutions on what are essentially social or psychic problems. Moreover, medical care is not a solution to society's problems of ill-health; to a large extent, medical care *is* the problem to which society is trying to find the solution. From this point of view, therefore, the NHS represents an attempt to solve problems which it is largely responsible for creating. It is not the intention of this section to explore in full the arguments of the new criticism. But, clearly, any assessment of the NHS must face the central challenge of these critics. This is the contention that the NHS has failed in what, after all, should be its overriding aim: to improve the people's health. What impact – if any – has the NHS had on the health of the people of Britain?

The question is horrendously difficult to answer. For any attempt to assess the NHS's impact on the population's state of health requires information about trends both before and after its creation. But there is only one reliable source of such information: mortality data. Death is a hard fact, which accommodates itself easily to statistical recording. So we know a great deal about what diseases people die of, and at what age. In contrast, we know remarkably little about how people live: the extent to which they suffer from non-threatening illnesses and the quality of their lives, and how this has changed over the years. The available statistics provide, at best, blurred snapshots rather than a clear moving picture over time. Moreover, the information is often extremely ambiguous. Take, for example, the well-documented upward trend in sickness absence in recent decades. This could be taken as evidence of growing ill-health in the population. But is it? It could, equally plausibly, be interpreted as an increasing willingness to take time off work: indeed there is evidence which shows, unsurprisingly, that if people are unhappy at work they are more likely to declare themselves sick.[34]

So, in effect, the available information permits statements only about the NHS's impact on how people die, not on how people live. In this respect, it is certainly difficult to show that the NHS has made much difference. Take, for instance, the case of infant mortality. This has fallen dramatically: from 43.7 per 1,000 births in 1947 to 16.1 in 1975.[35] But it is almost impossible to establish how much, if any, of this fall can be attributed to the NHS. Between 1930 and 1947, infant mortality also fell dramatically: from 67 to 43.7 per 1,000 births. The NHS, clearly, cannot take credit for that. Similarly, life expectancy has risen under the NHS. In 1948, a male child of one could expect to live for another 67.7 years. By the mid 1970s, the equivalent figure was 69.8. But, again, it is highly doubtful how much of the credit for this should go to the NHS. The evidence would seem to confirm the view that it is social and economic conditions – notable improvements in nutrition, housing and education – which promote health, as measured by such indicators as infant mortality or life expectancy, rather than an increasing capacity for medical intervention. International comparisons further reinforce this conclusion. For example, there seems to be no systematic relationship between the amount spent on health care in different countries and the various indicators of mortality. Britain spends a smaller proportion of a lower national income on health care than the United States or Germany, but does better than either on infant mortality and as well as both on life expectancy. On the other hand, Japan spends less than Britain, but does better on life expectancy and is only marginally worse on infant mortality.[36] One cross-national study has even found a statistical correlation between the number of doctors and mortality: the more doctors there are, the worse the mortality figures tend to be.[37]

Two, not necessarily contradictory, conclusions might be drawn from this evidence. The first is that different forms of health care provision – the way in which it is financed and organised – make no difference. The second is that, since it is impossible to demonstrate that spending money on health care makes any difference, the least spent the better: the facts would appear to support those who argue that medical intervention creates the problems which it is meant to solve. The case for the prosecution, as advanced by the new critics of health care, seems to be proved. Unfortunately the case for the prosecution rests on a fallacy. This is the assumption that *any* sensible conclusion about the performance of health services can be based exclusively on statistics of mortality. Granted that it is social and economic conditions which largely determine life expectancy and infant mortality, it is then both illogical and perverse to use these indicators to assess the performance of health services. For these tell us nothing about the contribution of the health service to the quality of the lives that are being extended or saved. If people live longer, they inevitably require more treatment for repair, maintenance and relief of such suffering as cannot be prevented. To assess the achievement of the NHS – or any other health service – we would therefore require information about its achievements in keeping an ageing population independent, active and mobile. But this, as pointed out previously, is precisely the kind of information that is lacking. 'The contribution of clinical services to health cannot be judged without statistics on such achievements', J. N. Morris has pointed out, 'and as we haven't the statistics we shouldn't make the judgements.'[38] All that the case for the prosecution has proved is that using inadequate statistics inevitably leads to drawing misleading conclusions.

What we do know, from the information about what the NHS actually does, is that a great many of its activities are designed precisely to improve the quality of life, as distinct from seeking to extend it. Every year, for example, some 100,000 people have eye operations to restore or maintain their sight. Every year, too, some 100,000 people have their hernias repaired. Every year, further, some 90,000 people have operations – such as plastic hip replacements – to stop them from becoming immobile cripples. None of these are conditions where people, if left untreated, would die – and so appear in the mortality statistics. All of these are conditions where, if they were neglected, the quality of people's lives would diminish greatly. The balance sheet is, of course, very complex. The NHS, doubtless, also extends some lives that have become a burden. Equally, the NHS does manufacture some social problems: for example, by keeping alive spina bifida and other severely handicapped babies who, in the past, would have died without benefit of medical intervention. But the picture drawn by some of the new critics – of a technological juggernaut intent only on preventing the inevitable approach of death, insensitive to both human and economic costs – is, clearly, an over-blown caricature.

To define the role of the NHS in terms of its contribution towards the quality of life, its capacity for caring for those who cannot be cured and its ability to minimise suffering, is to define the questions that should be asked, not to provide the answers. We simply do not know how many people who would have been permanently crippled with pain thirty-five years ago now lead more tolerable lives. We simply do not know how many people who would have been disabled thirty-five years ago can now lead normal lives. The information is irretrievable since we cannot resurrect the past. Nor do we know, though we are in a position to find out, how many people remain crippled or disabled whose conditions could, in fact, be alleviated: the long queue of people waiting to have plastic hip replacement surgery – a striking example of the contribution of technology to enhancing the quality of life – would suggest that there remains a considerable gap between what could be done, and what is being done. If there remains scope for disagreement about whether the NHS is doing enough to minimise human suffering – whether the appropriate balance has been struck between the priorities given to different forms of activity – we should at least be clear about the currency of evaluation that should be used in coming to any assessment of the NHS's achievements.

The new criticism, however, offers yet a further challenge to the concept on which the NHS is built. In accepting responsibility for minimising human suffering – in seeking to make more tolerable those conditions which cannot be cured by medical intervention – the NHS, it is argued, is playing an essentially repressive political role. To the extent that ill-health is generated by social or economic conditions, so the NHS becomes the servant of the *status quo* by making the consequences of those conditions more acceptable. By dealing with the symptoms of human suffering, it is in fact diverting attention from its causes: the medicalisation of social problems makes it that much easier for politicians to avoid addressing themselves to the underlying issues. So the NHS has become, if only involuntarily and unconsciously, an instrument for helping to shore up the existing distribution of power and wealth in society: a deceptively benevolent instrument of social control.

The point is incontrovertible but vacuous. Like all other social institutions, health services reflect the values of the society which has given birth to them. Like all other social institutions, too, health services are designed to provide an input of support to that society: a function which, as noted earlier in this chapter, the NHS performs admirably. To criticise the NHS (or any other health service) on the grounds that it is not an agent of social change but an agent of the *status quo* is therefore quite simply to miss the point. The NHS is – like the education system and like the judicial system – a device for maintaining the existing fabric of society, not for revolutionising it. It is, by its very nature, an established church: nonconformists and dissenters may, after all, opt out and set up their own conventicles of alternative medicine (the metaphor is more than a conceit: the supporters of alternative medicine resemble dissenters in so far as they reject medical authority and seek physical salvation through self-help).

But there is yet a further assumption in the new critique of the NHS, as an instrument of social control and political repression, which needs to be exposed and questioned. The point can be simply illustrated by taking an example much used by the new critics to demonstrate the futility, indeed the politically cosmetic nature, of much medical intervention. Every year, they point out, millions of tranquillisers are dished out to depressed housewives. But this is to deal only with the symptoms of distress, not with its causes. If housewives are depressed this may be because of poor housing, poverty or lack of job opportunities. Instead of helping them to adapt to a damaging or frustrating environment, it is argued, we should be acting to transform the environment itself. —

Again the point is incontrovertible but vacuous as a critique of the health care system. If doctors did not prescribe, if the suicide rate among depressed housewives suddenly leapt up, it does not follow that the political pressures for transforming the environment would become irresistible. Nor can it be taken for granted that, even if the political pressures for change were to become compelling, society would have the capacity to effect the necessary transformation. Social engineering is an uncertain art: many of the tranquillisers now being prescribed are part of the price being paid for previous experiments in social engineering, notably the attempt to remould the urban environment by tearing up established neighbourhoods and putting up tower blocks.

It would be misleading, however, to suggest that this faith in social engineering is the monopoly of the new criticism, although it may be its hallmark. It is shared by many who would reject outright the political analysis offered by the new criticism. Moreover, it represents a much more profound ideological challenge to the NHS than the ritualistic confrontations between the political parties. For the NHS is, in effect if not in intent, a monument to an ideology of original sin: it accepts the inevitability of ill-health and accordingly defines its role as being to deal with the consequences of circumstances over which it has no control. To assert an ideology of human perfectability – the belief that there is nothing inevitable about ill-health – is therefore to pose some fundamental questions both about its achievements and about its role: a point which is further explored in the next section.

FROM MEDICAL TO SOCIAL ENGINEERING

In the 1970s Britain, like the rest of the Western world, rediscovered prevention. The worldwide interest in prevention reflected both disillusionment and alarm. There was disillusionment with the capacity of medical science to produce health; medical science, it seemed, had reached the limits of its capacities to deliver technical solutions, such as vaccination or immunisation programmes, which actually prevented illness or disability. Its triumphs in delivering the world from such scourges as tuberculosis or polio lay in the past, seemingly; the new scourges such as cancer and heart disease appeared to be remarkably resistant to all the efforts of medical science to find a technological solution. Similarly, there was alarm about the relentless, apparently unstoppable increase in health care expenditure everywhere: giving medical science an open cheque on society's resources appeared to be a recipe for national bankruptcy.[39] So it is perhaps not surprising that the interest switched from medical engineering to social engineering in an attempt to devise ways of promoting good health, as distinct from providing services for dealing with ill-health.

Like the problems which provoked it, the interest was international. In 1974 the Canadian Government published what was to become the manifesto of the preventionists: the Lalonde report,[40] which set out the changes in environmental conditions and individual life-styles that might be expected to promote good health. In 1976 the British Government followed suit, publishing a discusion document setting out some of the policy options for prevention.[41] In 1977 a Sub-Committee of the Parliamentary Expenditure Committee took up the issue.[42] Its definition of how it saw its own task is worth quoting at some length since it illustrates many of the themes that recur in the debate about prevention:

The Sub-Committee felt it would be worthwhile to enquire to what extent and in which areas disease was being treated by the NHS where, with effective prevention within the limits of present knowledge, it need never have reached that stage. Effective prevention could in the long term free resources of medical skill, hospital beds and facilities to concentrate on diseases for which there are not at present any effective preventive measures. The Sub-Committee was particularly interested in the prevalence of disease precipitated by the individual's habits. Such diseases, sometimes described as 'diseases of civilisation' or 'self-induced' disease, include lung cancer, bronchitis and emphysema, which are usually caused by smoking, particularly cigarette smoking; coronary heart disease which is thought to be associated with a number of factors including smoking, particularly cigarette smoking, the Western-type diet rich in fat and refined foods including sugar, and the hardness of the water supply; obesity, and dental caries and gum disease whose development is at least encouraged by soft, sweet, sticky food; alcoholism and other harmful results of drinking too much and a number of other diseases of the intestines which may be due to an inadequate fibre intake. The incidence of many of these diseases appears to be increasing. One particularly distressing feature is that although to a greater or less extent preventable, most are not curable but can only be treated.

This definition illustrates both the width of the policy agenda and the complexity of the policy puzzles raised. Just how are people to be stopped from smoking cigarettes? Just how are they to be encouraged to adopt a healthier diet? Any answers to such questions involve a whole range of policy fields and policy tools. They range from persuasion through health education to regulation through the control of advertising, from increasing the taxes on damaging products to subsidising healthy products. Equally, they raise some prickly issues about the appropriate scope of public policy: about the extent to which government can legitimately limit the freedom of individuals to damage themselves (as distinct from damaging others).

But the scope and ambitions of a programme of prevention go further still. Prevention is not just about individual life styles; it is also about collective action. The two are inextricably linked, since the behaviour of individuals will be influenced by their social environment. Again the point is well illustrated by a quotation from the 1977 Parliamentary Committee report:

During the course of the enquiry it has been impressed on us repeatedly by the medical professions themselves that much of the most effective 'preventive medicine' is not within the scope of the National Health Service. In respect of individuals, for instance, the wearing of seat belts and crash helmets can save lives. From a community point of view, there is evidence that living in high-rise blocks is unsuitable for young families and elderly people; that firms employing fewer than 20 people have lower rates of sickness absence than larger organisations; that transport and planning policies which encourage people to take more exercise would be beneficial to health, and that the destruction of established communities by moving families to new estates instead of improving and conserving older houses where possible may lead to increased incidence of illness. To a considerable extent the NHS is expected to cope with the results of failures of policies in other fields.

To make prevention the first priority in health policy-making is thus to relegate the NHS to an almost peripheral role. Moreover the logic of prevention is the transformation of society. It suggests that the imperative of public policy should be the creation of an economy, a society and a working environment conducive to the production of good health as distinct from the production of ill-health. It is thus to introduce a new criterion into policy-making: to suggest that all policies should be assessed in terms of their contribution to the promotion of health. It is, furthermore, to question some of the existing criteria by which policies tend to be assessed. Thus it has been argued that if the production of health is our aim, then the production of extra wealth should take second place – since the emphasis on economic growth may, in itself, be a source of stress and ill-health in our society.[43] If health-effectiveness is the criterion, then cost-effectiveness may have to come second.

To adopt this approach is therefore to raise some very large questions. It raises some questions about the machinery of government. If the promotion of health involves every aspect of public policy – from taxation to town planning, from education to housing – then whose responsibility is it to co-ordinate the different departments involved and to devise a coherent programme of action? More crucially still, however, it raises questions about the political constituency for prevention. Supposing it were possible to devise a formal machinery of co-ordination (not a very difficult task), where would the political impetus for giving a health promotion bias to all public policies come from?

The NHS has, by the very fact of its existence, a political constituency: those whose income comes from working in it and those who, as patients, derive some direct benefits from its services. Prevention has no such constituency. Those who will benefit cannot be identified; moreover, the benefit itself is uncertain. For prevention is about the reduction of statistical risk, not about the delivery of certain benefits to specific individuals. The point was well made in the 1976 government report on prevention:

Statistical associations tell us very little about the size of the risk for any given individual. Many people with more than one of these undesirable attributes (i.e. obesity, lack of exercise, high blood pressure) never suffer heart attacks, at least up to an advanced age, while some people displaying none of these characteristics are struck down while still comparatively young.

In short, a policy of prevention will affect the lives of many people – a majority, indeed – who will not themselves benefit.

Here the contrast between the successful programmes of prevention in the past and the kind of measures now being advocated is instructive. The tradition of health promotion through social engineering is, of course, not new: it was the dominant approach in the nineteenth century. But the nineteenth century strategy delivered immediate benefits to large groups of the population: decent housing, clean water and efficient drains were desirable in themselves, quite apart from their contribution to improving the people's health. Present policies of prevention may, however, require people to accept what are perceived to be immediate disbenefits (higher taxes on cigarettes or alcohol, for example) in return for long term, contingent and uncertain benefits. It is precisely this imbalance between present costs and future benefits which explains the continuing frustration of the advocates of policies of prevention: the seemingly perverse reluctance of successive governments to adopt with any enthusiasm such self-evidently desirable policies.[44] The reason is simple. One man's political perversity is another man's political rationality. What is so self-evidently rational from the point of view of preventionists, is far less so from the perspective of the policy-makers. The costs of taking action, both political and economic, are paid in today's currency: if cigarette and alcohol consumption is cut, then factories will close down and workers will be declared redundant. Concentrated interests will be affronted; identifiable individuals will be injured. But the benefits, as already argued, will belong to the future and will, moreover, be diffuse and largely invisible. The inhibitions on political action thus outweigh the incentives: only appeals to paternalistic altruism are left. The expectations of the preventionists are thus destined to inevitable disillusion. If there are technical limitations on the capacity cf medical engineering to deliver the goods, so there are political limitations on the scope for social engineering. To invest total faith in either solution is to invite a sense of hopes betrayed.

The problems of social engineering are not only political, however. They reflect the difficulties both of mobilising a coalition for action and of devising appropriate policy tools. Furthermore, they may involve conflicts between different policy aims and values. The point can be illustrated by the case of the 1980 Black report on

'Inequalities in Health'[45]: the product of a research working group appointed by the Labour Government which submitted its recommendations to a Conservative administration. This report reached two main conclusions. First, it agreed that the inequalities in health between social classes had not been eliminated by the NHS.  Although everyone had gone up on the health escalator, the relative position of different socio-economic groups on it had not changed: thus, while infant mortality rates generally had dropped, the gap between social classes had remained. Second, the Black report concluded that these continuing differences were primarily attributable to social and economic conditions. It endorsed the thesis that: 'Whilst the health care services can play, and do play, a significant part in reducing inequalities in health, yet measures to reduce differences in material standards of living as experienced at work, in the home and in everyday social and community life are of even greater importance.' Its main recommendation followed from this diagnosis: a comprehensive anti-poverty strategy.

The strategy embodied an ambitious programme of social engineering. It called for the redistribution of income and the elimination of child poverty. It proposed an expanded programme of day care for children and comprehensive disablement allowances. It recommended improvements in working conditions and more spending on public housing. It envisaged the 'eventual phasing out of sales of harmful tobacco products at home and abroad'. Its message was, in short, that to transform the people's health also requires the transformation of society. Not surprisingly the Black report was rejected by a Conservative Government intent on trying to contain public expenditure. But it would have been equally surprising if it had been accepted by a Labour or Social Democrat Government. In the former case, the rejection was brutal and unsympathetic. In the latter case, the rejection would no doubt have been hand-wringing and apologetic. The reason lies not just in the fact that all governments grappling with a falling national income look askance at large demands for extra expenditure. It also lies in some of the assumptions built into the Black report: assumptions which explain why the social engineering approach so often appears to be inviting rejection.

The most important assumption made by the Black report was that the overriding, exclusive aim of policy should be the achievement of equality of outcome. That is, the success of policy should be measured by the extent to which it brought about not merely equality of access or equality of treatment within the NHS (see above) but equality in the distribution of health. It is not self-evident, however, that health policy can be based on a single value such as equality. Consider, an alternative aim of policy: to maximise the amount of health in the community. This is at least as plausible an objective as maximising equality. Yet the two conflict. The point can be simply illustrated. The Black report's objective of diminishing inequality could, for example, be achieved by scrapping all attempts to reduce cigarette smoking by means of health education campaigns. The evidence is that the upper social classes respond to such campaigns, while the lower social classes do not. The effect of attempts to improve the population's overall health, in this instance at least, is therefore to widen inequalities in its distribution. Abandon the attempt, and there will be greater equality – and more ill-health. So which aim of policy should have priority? Should the escalator be stopped, and the people on it moved nearer to each other, or should it be allowed to go on rising without any changes in the relative positions?

The dilemmas of policy, posed by the fact that there are competing aims, can be further illustrated. Take the case of infant mortality. Here there is, indeed, a disturbing difference between rates between the best-off and worst-off social groups. So an equality maximising strategy would concentrate on the worst-off: those in Social Class V. But it so happens that this class has been contracting. It now accounts for only 6 per cent of all births, as distinct from 20 per cent in 1931, although still contributing 11 per cent of all deaths. So a health maximising strategy would concentrate on those in Social Classes III and IV which between them contribute 63 per cent of all deaths.[46] Moreover, public policy might well have to ask itself which deaths cost least to prevent, and the answer might again be those in the higher social classes – who tend to be more influenced by health education and more accessible to medical intervention. In short, once more there is a direct collision between policies based on ethical imperatives (whether medical or egalitarian) and those based on utilitarian calculations, which take into account the opportunity costs of intervention: which ask questions about maximising the total benefits of policy rather than maximising the care given to individuals or single values.

It is precisely this neglect of opportunity costs – whether economic or political – which characterises the Black report's recommendations. Eradicating poverty and redistributing incomes may well be desirable policy aims in their own right. But as policy tools for improving the nation's health or equalising its distribution they are singularly blunt instruments. The relationship between living

176

* holding principle of equal rights for all people.

standards and health, as the report concedes, is a complex one: for instance, there are regional differences in health, cutting across social classes, which reflect other factors beside the distribution of income. So the case for embarking on the kind of ambitious programme of income redistribution and public expenditure recommended by the Black report rests, paradoxically, on the fact that we do not know precisely what are the determining socio-economic factors in promoting health.

Clearly, if a programme of social engineering is grandiose and comprehensive enough, then it will achieve at least some of its aims. But it will also be an extremely unappealing programme for policymakers who are conscious of cost constraints, and for whom improving the nation's health is only one of many policy aims all competing for scarce resources. Inherent in the social engineering approach to health policy is therefore the danger that, lacking a precise knowledge of the causal relationship between health and socio-economic conditions and, consequently, being unable to design specific policy tools, it will be driven to advocate general solutions on a scale which ensures their unacceptability and rejection.

BETWEEN UTOPIANISM AND NIHILISM

Assessing the performance of the NHS, this analysis would suggest, involves trying to discover a middle ground between utopianism and nihilism. To define the aims of the NHS in terms of the achievement of one overriding policy objective or value – whether the liquidation of ill-health or the elimination of inequality – is to set up utopian expectations which invite nihilistic disillusionment. This is why this chapter has, to return to the point made at the opening, sought to examine the performance of the NHS from different perspectives: using different currencies of evaluation leads to different figures at the end of the balance sheet. But inevitably each one of us will use a different exchange rate, based on our own values, as between the different currencies.

If the aim of the NHS is defined to be to eradicate disease and disability, then it is self-evidently a failure; if, however, its role is defined as being to minimise human suffering, then it can be reckoned as a reasonable success story. If the aim is defined to be to limit public expenditure, the NHS is a triumphant success story when measured against other health care systems in the Western world; if, in contrast, the aim is defined to be to maximise the total supply of health care, the NHS's performance is distinctly less impressive.

If the aim is defined to be to ration scarce resources in an equitable fashion, then the NHS is at least a comparative success story; if the aim is defined to be to achieve responsiveness to consumer demands, then the NHS fails to meet it.

In all this, to reiterate, the NHS represents an attempt to accommodate the conflicts between competing values and interests that characterise all pluralistic societies. It remains, as it began, a monument to political compromise. Its achievements have both been made possible by, and constrained by, the principle of political feasibility: the insistence on trying to contain conflict within consensus. It is this which explains the NHS's success as a political institution: it earns its keep in the political market place. It is this which explains the NHS's success as a functioning organisation, which defines problems in terms of its own capacity to deal with them rather than searching for ideal, but possibly unattainable, solutions. It is this, however, which also explains the dominance of organisational imperatives over other possible policy aims. It is this which explains the continuing tensions, the continuing search to reconcile what may be incompatible policy objectives, within the NHS. For to resolve the conflicts decisively – to choose between different aims and interests, instead of trying to reconcile them – might also end the consensus.

REFERENCES

1. DEPARTMENT OF HEALTH AND SOCIAL SECURITY, *Health and Personal Social Services Statistics for England, 1978*, HMSO: London 1980.
2. ROYAL COMMISSION ON THE CONSTITUTION, Research Paper no. 7, *Devolution and Other Aspects of Government: An Attitudes Survey*, HMSO: London 1973. See especially Table 38.
3. RICHARD TITMUSS, *The Gift Relationship*, Allen & Unwin: London 1970.
4. COMMISSION OF THE EUROPEAN COMMUNITIES, *The Perception of Poverty in Europe*, EEC: Brussels 1977.
5. For a review of the available evidence, see Vivienne Walters, *Class, Inequality and Health Care*, Croom Helm: London 1980, and Peter Townsend, 'Inequality and the Health Service', *The Lancet*, 15 June 1974, pp. 1179–89. For a somewhat different interpretation, see Elizabeth Collins and Rudolf Klein, 'Equity and the NHS: Self-Reported Morbidity, Access and Primary

Care', *British Medical Journal*, 25 Oct. 1980, pp. 1111–15.

6. RICHARD TITMUSS, *Commitment to Welfare*, Allen & Unwin: London 1968.

7. L. A. ADAY and ROBERT EICHHORN, *The Utilization of Health Services: Indices and Correlates – A Research Bibliography*, U.S. Department of Health, Education and Welfare: Washington, D.C. 1972.

8. SOCIAL SERVICES COMMITTEE, Third Report, Session 1980–81, *Public Expenditure on the Social Services*, HMSO: London 1981, H. C. 324, vol, 11, pp. 12–14.

9. DEPARTMENT OF HEALTH AND SOCIAL SECURITY, *Hospital In-Patient Enquiry, 1977*, HMSO: London 1980. This is the source for the subsequent statistics of NHS activity quoted in this chapter.

10. MARTIN BUXTON and RUDOLF KLEIN, *Allocating Health Resources*, Royal Commission on the National Health Service, Research Paper no. 3, HMSO: London 1978.

11. JOHN R. BUTLER, *Family Doctors and Public Policy*, Routledge & Kegan Paul: London 1973.

12. BUXTON and KLEIN, *op. cit.*

13. RUDOLF KLEIN, 'Policy Options for Medical Manpower', *British Medical Journal*, 9 July 1977, pp. 136–7; Alan Maynard and Arthur Walker, 'A Critical Survey of Medical Manpower Planning in Britain', *Social and Economic Administration*, vol. 11, no. 1, Spring 1977, pp. 52–75.

14. ROYAL COMMISSION on the National Health Service, *Report*, HMSO: London 1979, Cmnd. 7615.

15. BRIAN ABEL-SMITH, 'Minimum Adequate Levels of Personal Health Care: History and Justification', *Milbank Memorial Fund Quarterly / Health and Society*, vol. 56, no. 1, Winter 1978, pp. 7–22. The issue contains a number of other articles bearing on the theme of minimum adequate levels.

16. PETER A. WEST, *The Nation's Health and the NHS*, King's Fund Centre: London 1980.

17. LEE DONALDSON ASSOCIATES, *UK Private Medical Care: Provident Schemes Statistics, 1980*, Lee Donaldson Associates: London 1981.

18. RUDOLF KLEIN, 'Is There a Case For Private Practice?', *British Medical Journal*, 6 Dec. 1975, pp. 59–3.

19. ROYAL COMMISSION ON THE NATIONAL HEALTH SERVICE, Research Paper no. 5, *Patients' Attitudes to the Hospital Service*, HMSO: London 1978.

20. CONSUMERS ASSOCIATION, *Children in Hospital*, Consumers Association: London 1980.
21. This analysis is based on the model developed by A. O. Hirschman, *Exit, Voice and Loyalty*, Harvard U. P.: Cambridge, Mass., 1970. See also Rudolf Klein, 'Models of Man and Models of Policy: Reflections on *Exit, Voice and Loyalty*', *Milbank Memorial Fund Quarterly / Health and Society*, vol. 58, no. 3, Summer 1980, pp. 416–29.
22. A. H. BIRCH, 'Economic Models in Political Science: The case of *Exit, Voice and Loyalty*', *British Journal of Political Science*, vol 5, 1975, pp. 62–72,
23. ARTHUR SELDON (ed.), *The Litmus Papers: A National Health Dis-service*, Centre for Policy Studies: London 1980.
24. T. R. MARMOR and JAMES A. MORONE, 'Representing Consumer Interests: Imbalanced Markets, Health Planning and the HSAs', *Milbank Memorial Fund Quarterly / Health and Society*, vol. 58, no. 1, Winter 1980, pp. 125–65.
25. COMMITTEE OF INQUIRY INTO THE REGULATION OF THE MEDICAL PROFESSION, *Report*, HMSO: London 1975, Cmnd. 6018.
26. GENERAL MEDICAL COUNCIL, *Annual Report*, London 1981.
27. RUDOLF KLEIN, with the assistance of Ann Howlett, *Complaints Against Doctors*, Charles Knight: London 1973.
28. HEALTH SERVICE COMMISSIONER, *Annual Report, 1980–81*, HMSO: London 1981, H. C. 368.
29. SELECT COMMITTEE ON THE PARLIAMENTARY COMMISSIONER FOR ADMINISTRATION, First Report, Session 1977–78, *Independent Review of Hospital Complaints in the National Health Service*, HMSO: London 1977, H. C. 45.
30. See, for example, the leading article 'Towards Medical Audit', *British Medical Journal*, 16 Feb. 1974, pp. 255–7, and the symposium of papers on this theme in the same issue.
31. DEPARTMENT OF HEALTH AND SOCIAL SECURITY, *Report on Confidential Enquiries into Maternal Deaths in England and Wales, 1967–1969*, HMSO: London 1972.
32. COMMITTEE OF ENQUIRY: MEDICAL PROFESSION IN THE UNITED KINGDOM, *Competence to Practice*, London 1976 (no publisher given).
33. For a scholarly source, on which much of the new criticism is based, see Thomas McKeown, *The Role of Medicine*, Nuffield Provincial Hospitals Trust: London 1976. For a popular conflation of the ideas of the new criticism, see Ian Kennedy, *The Unmasking of Medicine*, Allen & Unwin: London 1981. Also see

Ivan Illich, *Limits to Medicine*, Penguin: Harmondsworth 1977.

34. OFFICE OF HEALTH ECONOMICS, *Sickness Absence: A Review*, OHE Briefing no. 16: London, August 1981.

35. PETER WEST, *op. cit.*

36. ROYAL COMMISSION ON THE NATIONAL HEALTH SERVICE, *Report, op cit.*

37. A. L. COCHRANE, A. S. ST. LEGER AND F. MOORE, 'Health Service "Input" and Mortality "Output" in Developed Countries', *Journal of Epidemiology and Community Health*, vol. 7, no. 2, June 1978, pp. 200–206.

38. J. N. MORRIS, 'Are Health Services Important to the People's Health?', *British Medical Journal*, 19 Jan. 1980, pp. 167–8.

39. The literature on the explosion of health care costs is vast. But see, for example, D. A. Ehrlich (ed.), *The Health Care Cost Explosion*, Hans Huber: Bern 1975; Robert Maxwell, *Health Care: The Growing Dilemma*, McKinsey: New York 1975.

40. M. A. LALONDE, *New Perspectives on the Health of Canadians*, Canadian Department of National Health and Welfare: Ottawa 1974.

41. DEPARTMENT OF HEALTH AND SOCIAL SECURITY, *Prevention and Health: Everybody's Business*, HMSO: London 1976.

42. EXPENDITURE COMMITTEE, First Report, Session 1976–77, *Preventive Medicine*, HMSO: London 1977, H. C. 169.

43. PETER DRAPER, GORDON BEST AND JOHN DENNIS, *Health, Money and the National Health Service*, Unit for the Study of Health Policy, Guy's Hospital: London 1976.

44. See, for example, the editorial, 'The Avoidable Holocaust', *British Medical Journal*, 5 April 1980, pp. 959–60.

45. DEPARTMENT OF HEALTH AND SOCIAL SECURITY, Report of a Research Working Group, *Inequalities in Health*, DHSS: London 1980.

46. RAYMOND ILLSLEY, *Professional or Public Health?*, Nuffield Provincial Hospitals Trust: London 1980.

Chapter six
POSSIBLE FUTURES: THE VIEW IN 1983

Only one prediction can be made with absolute confidence about the future of the NHS. This is that it will continue to generate more demands on the political economy. From an international, comparative perspective, the NHS may appear to be a remarkably efficient machine for containing consumer demands.[1] Whatever the statistics about the distribution of resources may say, the perceived equity of the British health service appears to make rationing and scarcity acceptable. From a national perspective, however, the NHS is a political organisation for mobilising and articulating demands: its one million workers make it perhaps the most formidable lobby in the country pressing for extra funds.

Moreover, in the 1980s the antithesis between the ability of the NHS to control consumer demands and its role in articulating producer demands is no longer as neat as it was in the immediate decades after its creation. As the two previous chapters have shown, the opening up of the arena of health care policy has brought on stage not only new groups of producers but also lobbies speaking for client groups. Both the political and the private market of health care have expanded: an expansion which, in both cases, reflects the pressure of unsatisfied demands. The point is further reinforced by the very nature of health care. Even if the limitations of medical technology in curing disease and disability are now becoming apparent, there are no such limitations on the scope of health services for providing care for those who cannot be cured. Even if policies of prevention and social engineering were to be successfully introduced, their very success in extending life expectancy would create new demands for alleviating the chronic degenerative diseases of old age. In short, no policy can ensure that people will drop dead painlessly at the age of 80, not having troubled the health services previously.

The demands being generated by the NHS, however, are political as well as economic. Again, the implications of an exploding health care policy arena require to be stressed. With more actors involved in the policy arena, with the frequent inability of the traditional corporate organisations such as the BMA to deliver the goods, the actual process of decision-making has become more complex and difficult. In short, the political costs of getting things done in the arena of health care policy are rising as, to revert to a point emphasised earlier, more groups are able to impose delays or to veto change. If there can be certainty about the inevitability of increasing demands, we have to reach for the crystal ball when considering the other side of the equation: the capacity (and willingness) of the political system to respond to the demands generated from within the health care policy arena. Here there are two sets of uncertainties which have to be taken into account: the performance of the economy and the ideological bias of whatever government happens to be in office. While the performance of the economy will determine the political costs of meeting the health care demands, it is the ideological bias of the government which is likely to shape the precise response.

Let us first look at the implications of making optimistic assumptions about the future of the British economy. If we assume a resumption of the growth rates that characterised the economy until the mid-1970s – low by comparison with other Western countries but high by Britain's own historical standards – then the extra demands generated by the health care policy arena could be financed, relatively painlessly, out of the dividends of growth. There would be no need to choose between permitting the continued expansion of the NHS, and other public services, and allowing private consumption to rise. Both could go on increasing: the pattern of the 1960s and the early 1970s. In such circumstances, it would seem reasonable to assume also that there might be no great pressures for a radical change in the present system of health care: change could be expected to be gradual, adaptive and incremental, in line with the experience since 1948. The emphasis would be on solving some of the inherited problems and accommodating some of the emerging pressures, rather than on going back to the drawing board. Conflict would continue to be contained within consensus.

Now, however, let us look at the implications of making more pessimistic – and, alas, probably also more realistic – assumptions about the future of the British economy. If we assume a continuation of the trends established since the mid-1970s, if we think that the

British economy will at best veer between long periods of stagnation and short bursts of growth, then the extra demands generated by the health care policy arena will present governments with a problem for which there is no painless solution. To maintain the present system of health care would also be to accept the political costs of financing it out of taxation (or, which comes to the same thing in terms of reducing people's pay packets, out of national insurance contributions). There would be direct competition between the claims of the NHS and the claims of private consumption. Moreover, continuing high unemployment would almost certainly reinforce the demands on the NHS: while the evidence as to whether unemployment actually causes ill-health is as yet inconclusive, there can be no doubt that it lowers the time costs of those involved. If you are out of work, you have by definition more time to queue in the doctor's surgery. In such circumstances it would seem reasonable to assume an increasing readiness to question the very nature of the present system of health care: a break with the experience since 1948. The trends towards ideological polarisation, which became apparent during the second half of the 1970s, might intensify; increasing conflict might break the mould of consensus.

So much for the general considerations which are likely to affect the future debate about the NHS and health care policy. In what follows, this chapter examines some of the specific policy options that are available to deal not only with the inherited problems of the NHS, which have provided the subject matter of previous chapters, but also with the new problems which will be created if the pessimistic assumptions about the British economy turn out to be accurate. The aim of this exercise is to display the range of possible futures for the NHS and the organisation of health care, not to evaluate them in detail: to show the menu from which the political parties are likely to choose, not to provide a good food guide. For, to recapitulate a theme which has run through this book, health care policy-making involves a choice between competing and conflicting policy aims, and the nature of that choice must inevitably depend on the value systems of ideologies of those making them.

Table 1 therefore sets out, in summary form, the various policy aims and values that are invoked in debates about health care policy: drawing on the discussions in previous chapters. The first column presents the core aims and values of the traditional NHS assumptive world. The second column presents those of the NHS's critics who challenge not the collectivist provision of health services, or the

Table 1 Policy aims and values in health care

NHS	Collectivist critics	Market critics
Equity in the distribution of services	Equality of out come (social engineering)	Individual choice
Efficiency		
Expertise	Consumer participation	Consumer sovereignty
Rationing by need		Responding to demand
Bureaucratic rationality	Anti-bureaucratic	Anti-bureaucratic
National standards	Localism	Pluralism
	Worker participation	
Minimising tax burden	Minimising demands (prevention)	Maximising people's willingness to pay for own care

financial basis of the present system, but existing organisational forms and policy priorities. The final column presents those of the NHS's market critics who challenge the collectivist provision of health services, and argue for a switch to an insurance-financed system. In what follows we shall discuss future policy options in terms of the trade-offs both between, and within, these three categories.[2]

Taking the existing framework of the NHS, and the inherited pattern of perceptions and assumptions, the traditional response to an imbalance between demands and resources would be to impose greater bureaucratic rationality: to try to squeeze more out of what is available by increasing efficiency. In this respect, we find the rhetoric of the early 1980s echoing that of the early 1950s: in both periods, an efficiency drive was the response to financial stringency. The logic of continued stringency would be to move from exhortation to bureaucratic control: to insist that the professional providers of services should be accountable to the bureaucracy for the way in which they use resources. It would be to introduce a system of public audit of medical practice designed to make consultants and general practitioners answerable for the way in which they use beds or prescribe drugs.

To make this point is also to suggest that, in practice, the problem of reconciling rising demands and stagnant resources cannot be solved simply by asserting bureaucratic rationality. Political logic does not support economic logic. The political costs of any move which would threaten medical autonomy, by introducing an element of bureaucratic control, have so far inhibited all governments, and there is little reason to expect any change in future. Moreover, as the previous chapters have argued, the problem of control stems from the fact that there are no agreed national norms of practice. The paradox would seem to be that only the medical profession could develop such norms, and it is difficult to see why it should seek to develop tools of accountability which would subordinate it to the bureaucracy: the principle (or fiction) of infinite diversity is the essential safeguard of medical autonomy.

So it is not surprising that the present government has moved in the direction of both blame-diffusion and demand-diffusion by respectively invoking the values of localism and encouraging the development of the private market. Both represent policies for lessening the demands on central government. While the encouragement of the private market might be ideologically unacceptable to a government dedicated to maintaining a universal NHS, the move towards localism would remain in an attractive policy option: decentralisation appears to meet the demands of the collectivist critics for greater consumer participation and to respond to their suspicion of bureaucracy. It is less clear, though, whether the decentralisation option is compatible with maintaining the achievement of equity in the distribution of services as the dominant aim of policy. If, in fact, more decisions are to be taken at the periphery and if there is to be less bureaucratic control over the way in which resources are used locally, then this implies the acceptance of more diversity.[3] Once more we are back to the original dilemma of the NHS: the trade-off between seeking to achieve national standards (which implies centralisation) and local autonomy.

While the dilemma is as old as the NHS itself, however the political and economic environment in which it is being discussed has changed. If blame-diffusion and demand-diffusion are indeed going to become the policy themes of the 1980s, then the policy options rejected in 1946 may become more attractive: specifically, the option of transferring responsibilty for health services to local government may once again appear on the policy agenda. If diversity is inevitable anyway – since the costs of achieving national uniformity are too great – why not make a virtue of necessity? Why not embrace the values of localism whole-heartedly? One reason against doing so is the political cost involved: the medical profession's opposition to local government control has not diminished since 1948, and is shared by other health service providers. Additionally, there are some practical problems. It is quite clear that the present rate-based system of local government finance could not cope with the burden of health services: either these would have to be financed directly by central government, so limiting the scope of local autonomy, or a new method of raising local revenues would have to be devised. Again, local government boundaries were not designed with health services in mind: a problem aggravated, but not caused, by the 1982 reorganisation of the NHS which scrapped the principle of co-terminosity. Nor is it self-evident that local government control can be equated with greater consumer participation, or less bureaucracy. The case of education would seem to offer a warning example on this point: local government control has not diminished demands for greater public involvement in the running of schools, for instance.

The logic of localism points, however, to a more radical policy option still. This is that of transferring control over health services to elected local bodies. What could be simpler than to make the members of the District Health Authorities directly elected, rather than nominated? Would this not be to institutionalise the principle of local democracy? Central government could still allocate the funds through some system of block grants, so ensuring distributional justice in the allocation of resources. The elected bodies would be responsible for the way in which the funds were spent: a degree of diversity would be the inevitable price to be paid for conceding them autonomy.

Again, some problems need to be noted. First, such a solution would re-open the debate about the relative merits of all-purpose elected authorities, as distinct from specially elected functional bodies. If there were to be specially elected health authorities, why not apply the same principle to education? Why not, indeed, may be the answer, but this once more suggests that fundamental changes in the administration of health care may presuppose fundamental changes in the existing system of delivering local services as a whole. Second, more centrally still, on present evidence it seems highly doubtful whether voters would support the principle of local democracy in health care by actually turning out to vote. The experience of local government is not encouraging: yet in the case of health services the incentives to turn out to vote are even less than in the case of local government services. As was noted earlier, use is contingent on people falling ill (in contrast to such services as refuse collection or street lighting where we obtain information about their efficiency and effectiveness by the mere fact of being local residents). The experience of New Zealand is not encouraging either; local health authorities were directly elected and apathy was the norm.[4] Local involvement would almost certainly be in a direct relationship to the degree of autonomy enjoyed by health authorities: the incentives to take part in local political activity would rise as their freedom to diverge from national patterns increased. Furthermore, to revert to the earlier discussion of political markets, local control might reinforce the bias towards the acute services at the expense of the most vulnerable and deprived groups: those groups least likely to be able to press their own interests.

Nor is it self-evident that local democracy would necessarily be a successful instrument for asserting the voice of the consumer against the voice of the expert. If the problems of controlling professional expertise have not so far been solved in the context of the NHS, it is difficult to see why in future part-time elected members should succeed where full-time administrators have failed. To the extent that these problems arise from an imbalance of information – from the fact that professional providers are perceived to have the right of defining both needs and appropriate responses – it is difficult to see what difference will result from replacing nominated by elected members. The success of teachers in guarding the contents of the curriculum from lay scrutiny, referred to in the previous chapter, would seem to suggest that it is the imbalance of organised power and knowledge between service producers and service consumers which is the decisive factor, rather than the institutional context of the service concerned. If it is the professionals who largely shape consumer expectations and perceptions of what is possible and desirable, then the paradox of local democracy may be to give more power to the local producers – emancipated from the paternalistic rationalisers who, in the context of the national health care policy, provide a source of counter-expertise and assert values which may run contrary to those of both local producers and local consumers.

To accept the inevitability of producer dominance suggests yet a further policy option. If the reality of any health service is that it will be dominated by its producers, why not institutionalise the fact of worker syndicalism? Why not translate the present veto powers of the producers into a positive responsibility for providing health care? Framed in these terms, the questions would seem to point towards a Yugoslav solution: the transfer of all NHS facilities – hospitals, health centres and so on – to worker co-operatives: so fulfilling G. D. H. Cole's vision of health services being run by guilds of self-governing workers, based on small units 'so that the initiative of individual medical men, or groups of fellow-workers, may not be hampered by too much central control'.[5] Ironically, it would seem that *realpolitik*, in terms of recognising where power really lies, marches hand in hand with political radicalism: that accepting producer dominance may be the price to be paid for decentralisation, encouraging local initiative and freedom from bureaucracy.

Once again, one man's policy solution is another man's policy problem. Even assuming that the health service workers could agree as to just how they would run such co-operatives (a large assumption, given the internal rivalries and the claim of the medical profession to a commanding role), there remains the question of who would decide what health services should be produced. After all, no one would dream of giving the producers an open cheque to decide their own priorities and to determine what services should be available to whom. The solution favoured by the original Guild Socialists appears to have been some form of negotiated contract between guilds of producers and guilds of consumers. Similarly, it is possible to conceive of such contracts being negotiated by either central or local government, specifying what they wanted by way of services, and then leaving it to the producers to decide how best to provide them. But, paradoxically, what appears to be the most radically left-wing policy option is also entirely consistent with what is usually considered to be the most right-wing policy option: a return to a market system where individuals buy their own health care (see the third column, Table 1). If co-operatives of health care producers are to be made responsive to consumer demands – instead of pursuing their own self-interests – then clearly a market system would seem to be the best answer: if the co-operatives did not provide the services wanted by the customers, they would go bankrupt.

To make this point is to underline the fact that to advocate a market system of health care is not synonymous with advocating a *private* market system, nor does it necessarily involve relying on the profit principle. A clear distinction requires to be drawn between the organisation of health care and its financing, between the ownership of the actual physical resources and the way in which they are paid for. So far the discussion of policy options has been in terms of organisation only: the assumption has been that while the organisation of health services may change, the method of financing them will not. If, however, we consider different methods of finance, a new set of policy options becomes available. For example, one option might be to leave the NHS organisationally intact, but to introduce a universal system of health insurance. Under such a system the NHS would recoup its costs by charging for services rendered, instead of being financed out of taxation by means of central government budgeting. Alternatively, the NHS might, under such a system, simply become one of a number of different institutions, public, private or non-profit making, competing for custom: its size being determined by its ability to respond to consumer demands.

It is, clearly, possible to have a system of health care which covers the entire population without also having a universal health service. If the State makes health insurance compulsory for all citizens – and if, further, the State also pays the health care contributions of whose who lack the means and of those whose handicaps are so severe that no insurance scheme could cover the costs – then there is no reason of principle why such a scheme should not provide the same comprehensive coverage as the NHS. But, equally clearly, there are a number of difficulties.[6] To the extent that the State makes such a scheme mandatory, so insurance contributions may simply be seen as another form of taxation: thereby defeating the political objective of reducing the government's revenue-raising role. Moreover, insurance creates rights to benefits: it entitles consumers to make certain demands. In contrast to the NHS, it thus gives political visibility to the problem of rationing. It would immediately raise such questions as whether there was to be a universal entitlement to renal dialysis or plastic hip replacement (to revert to some of the examples of rationing in the NHS discussed earlier). If yes, then obviously the cost of providing health care would rise: one of the arguments of the advocates of a market system is precisely that Britain is spending less collectively on health care than its inhabitants individually would be prepared to pay. But universal rights would legitimise the demands not only of those with the capacity to pay but also of those for whom the State would be picking up the bill: and since something like 50 per cent of the NHS's resources are devoted to the elderly, this would suggest that the Government's residual financial obligations would continue to be heavy. If, however, the answer is no – if there are not to be such universal entitlements – then we are back to the issue of equity: if there is to be a hierarchy of entitlements, what criteria will be used to decide who gets what?

Once more a paradox requires noting. Just as the seemingly left-wing syndicalist option would seem to be most consistent with the apparently right-wing market option, so in turn the market option would seem to require a radically egalitarian income redistribution policy to satisfy the equity criterion. For if demand is to decide who gets what – as distinct from professionally determined need – then the equity criterion would require that the capacity to make such demands should be distributed in an inverse ratio to people's state of health: income would have to be re-distributed to the least healthy. The real question then becomes whether it is politically more feasible to redistribute resources through the machinery of the NHS than to redistribute income through the machinery of taxation. To put the question in this form is to suggest, perhaps, that this would be to replace a merely difficult aim of policy with a wholly impossible one. If it is the healthy who tend to have the most power in the economic market, the same applies in the case of the political market. So the conclusion would seem to be that, whatever the advantages or disadvantages of the market option, it does imply a trade-off between the policy aim of maximising the resources devoted to health care and that of achieving distributional equity. If in theory the two are reconcilable, in practice they would seem to diverge.

There are, however, a number of further policy options for reducing the demands on the public sector by privatising the problem of health care, while still maintaining the present institutional and financial structure of the NHS. At present the NHS has, in effect, an open-ended commitment to deal with the production of ill-health by the socio-economic system: it takes on the problems of cure and care which are generated by society at large. However, it is possible to conceive of strategies which would attempt to reverse this process and, by doing so, to limit the demands on the NHS. One policy option is to redefine medical as social problems: the de-medicalisation of health care. Such a strategy would seek to push the burden of care onto the family and the community. The trend in this direction has been apparent in Britian for the past two decades, under both Conservative and Labour governments, and it has been justified in terms of both cost-effectiveness and humanitarianism: non-institutional care, it is argued, is not only cheaper but also more humane for those concerned. Moreover, it fits in snugly with the revolt against expertise and bureaucracy: the invocation of self-help and voluntary action cuts across ideological divides by appealing to the values of both individualism and community solidarity.

Although the case for this option is often presented in terms of

its ability to reduce the costs of health care, its real appeal is somewhat different. It is that the costs are carried by the private sector
rather than by the public sector. The burden on families of providing care for elderly relatives or handicapped children is no less real
for not appearing in the national accounts, and for being difficult to
translate into money terms. The political acceptability of such an
option may therefore depend crucially on its political visibility:
whether or not people see through it.

The option also implies an ability to reverse what would appear
to be a deep-rooted social trend. If the growth of demands on the
NHS reflects, in part at least, the externalisation of caring services
previously provided in the home then this, in turn, would seem to
reflect a major social revolution: the increasing participation of
women in the labour force. To a large extent it can be argued that
many of the women employed in the NHS are carrying out precisely
the same kind of job – domestic household chores and the basic caring routines for patients – which they previously might have carried
out in their own homes. If this is so, then any attempt to reverse
this trend has profound implications for the distribution of income
and for the distribution of work between the sexes. Moreover, at a
time of high unemployment, there would seem to be a strong argument for using the NHS as a job-creating programme[7]: for increasing
the number of less skilled jobs – the jobs of those primarily engaged
in the caring role – while reducing the numbers of the more expensive skilled professionals. But such a policy for developing the caring
function of the NHS, by a deliberate process of changing the balance
of skills employed, would run counter to the policy option of seeking
to privatise the burden of care. Again we are faced by a conflict
between different aims of policy.

The other policy option available for limiting the demands on the
NHS is to make those responsible for generating ill-health pay the
costs involved: to reverse the process whereby the collective provision of health care relieves the producers of ill-health from the financial consequence of their activities. This is indeed the logic of past
policies for regulating health and safety in industry. It would also
be the logic of making the provision of occupational health schemes
compulsory. Once again the argument for such an option would be
that it would transform public into private costs. But in contrast to
the option for transforming public into private costs by transferring
the burden of care to the family and the community, this one challenges the interests of an organised and concentrated political constituency. The point is well illustrated by the experience of the

Conservative Government when, in 1981, it sought to privatise the public costs of social security payments for sickness absence by transferring responsibility to employers.[8] The rationale for such a move was strong, quite apart from the savings to the Government: by making employers responsible for sickness absence payments, it would also give them a direct incentive to improve those workplace conditions which caused ill-health. In the outcome, however, the resistance of the employers forced the Government to make compensatory financial concessions to industry on such a scale as to negate the original hope of actually saving money. If economic recession strengthens the arguments for reducing the demands on the public sector, it also reinforces the resistance of industry to any measures which increase its costs and decrease its competitiveness in the international market place.

Perhaps only one conclusion can safely be drawn from this brief review of some of the possible policy options. This is that Britain is likely to move towards a more pluralistic system of health care. For if the politics of the NHS over the past thirty-five years demonstrate anything, it is that there is no way of reconciling all the various interests, all the various competing policy aims and values that are inevitably and inextricably involved in the health care policy arena. This is why the history of the NHS is so very largely a history of different attempts to address the same problems: why the previous chapters have told the story of policy making as a continuing dialogue about the same, recurring themes. From this perspective the NHS is an institution which internalises and reflects tensions and conflicts inevitable in a pluralistic society.

To the extent that those tensions and conflicts are themselves constrained by an overarching social and political consensus, so they are also containable within the NHS. This was, indeed, the pattern until the 1980s. But to the extent that the demands on the political and economic system rise faster than its capacity to satisfy them, so it becomes more imperative to diffuse tensions and to decentralise conflict. Institutions like the NHS which once were a proud monument to national consensus can, in these circumstances, all too easily become an embarrassing monument to national failure. This would suggest that the role of the NHS will become less dominant in future: that the trends towards a mixed economy of health care and towards a more loosely articulated system will continue. For while it is important to recognise the reality of ideological conflict, it is equally significant that the different ideological languages are to a large extent delivering the same message: less bureaucracy, less centralisation and less deference to professional expertise, more self-help, more consumer participation and more tolerance of diversity. While there are sharp divergences about the policy means for achieving these aims – and about what other valued objectives should or should not be sacrificed in the process – there is a remarkable degree of agreement about the general direction of desirable change.

REFERENCES

1. ROBERT MAXWELL, *Health and Wealth*, Lexington: Lexington, Mass. 1981.
2. My discussion of policy options draws on a conference paper written jointly with Celia Davies: while she would no doubt disagree with some of the conclusions drawn, the analysis leans on her contribution.
3. RUDOLF KLEIN, 'Control, Participation and the British National Health Service', *Milbank Memorial Fund Quarterly / Health and Society*, vol. 57, no. 1, Winter 1979, pp. 70–95.
4. MINISTRY OF HEALTH, *A Health Service for New Zealand*, Government Printer: Wellington 1974.
5. G. D. H. COLE, *Guild Socialism Re-Stated*, Leonard Parsons: London 1920.
6. ALAN MAYNARD, 'Pricing, Insurance and the National Health Service', *Journal of Social Policy*, vol. 8, no. 2, April 1979, pp. 157–76.
7. SOCIAL SERVICES COMMITTEE, Third Report, Session 1980–81, *Public Expenditure on the Social Services*, HMSO: London 1981, H.C. 324.
8. MICHAEL O'HIGGINS, 'Income During Initial Sickness: An Analysis and Evaluation of a New Strategy for Social Security', *Policy and Politics*, vol. 9, no. 2, April 1981, pp. 151–71.

Chapter seven
THE POLITICS OF MODERNISATION: EVENTS, 1983–1989

At the start of 1989 it is possible, depending on one's perspective, to make two quite contradictory statements about the National Health Service both of which, however, happen to be true. Taking a long distance view of the NHS, it is an island of stability in a sea of turbulent change. A Conservative Government which prides itself on its iconoclasm about almost every British institution and which has shown itself hostile to the interest groups guarding the status quo, has just published a Review[1] that confirms the special status of the NHS as a protected species. The principle of a tax-financed, universal, free at the point of delivery health care system, established in 1948, has been re-affirmed despite pressure to abandon it. The institution stands; the threatening waves have receded. Yet looking at the institution from the inside, as it were, the NHS is in a process of change unprecedented in its history: a process which will be accelerated by the Government's Review. There has been a dislocation of inherited conventions and practices, as well as subtle shifts in the internal balance of power, that have created a sense both of insecurity and of new possibilities. What we have, then, is the picture of an institution where, behind the stately facade, the workmen are beginning to gut the old building. The politics of the NHS in the 1980s can thus be read as the story of adaptation to a new environment in a situation where change is constrained by organisational coalitions and public loyalties forged over the previous 40 years.

In analysing the NHS's new environment, it is helpful to distinguish between underlying social, economic and technological trends and the way in which Mrs Thatcher's Government has chosen to respond to the resulting challenge of change. The trends themselves, of course, largely reflect slow movements in the glacier over decades. So, for example, the transformation of the British economy from its dependence on the traditional heavy industries to a service economy heavily reliant on information technology has been long in the making,[2] and is still far from complete. It is the sharpness of the perception of change, the growing awareness that a new kind of society was (for better or worse) emerging from the ruins of Britain's 19th century industrial legacy, that increasingly marked the decade as it progressed towards its end: the emergence of a new intellectual climate. It was a transformation reflected in the politics of the 1980s: the only period in Britain's 20th century history where one Government will (barring a miracle) have been in power for an entire decade without interruption. For the 1980s have been remarkable both for the domination of Mrs Thatcher and for the attempts of other parties to re-think their own styles and policies: the growing awareness, in the Labour as well as in the centre parties, that a new environment calls for a new kind of politics. Hence the importance of not interpreting the politics of the NHS (or indeed of any other policy area) simply in terms of the ideological preferences or idiosyncracies of Mrs Thatcher's Administration but of seeing them also as the product of the forces which put her, and kept her, in office in the 1980s.[3]

THE CHANGING ENVIRONMENT

The NHS was born into a working class society only slowly emerging from war, where rationing and queueing were symbols not of inadequacy but of fairness in the distribution of scarce resources. It celebrated its 40th anniversary in 1988 in what had become an affluent consumer society, where only access to work was rationed. Whereas in 1951 over 64 per cent of the occupied population were manual workers, by 1981 the proportion had fallen to fewer than 48 per cent. Whereas in 1947, only 27 per cent of the population owned their own homes, by 1981 the proportion had risen to 58 per cent.[4] It is a society, therefore, where an increasing number of people take it for granted that they control their own lives. It is a society, too, whose politics are marked by diminishing partisanship and an increasing willingness to shop around among the parties; even the proportion of voters identifying with the Conservatives has fallen.[5] Brand loyalty cannot be taken for granted and support, increasingly, depends on perceptions of performance.

It would be a mistake, however, to imply that Britain has moved into the era of the politics of private consumption, dominated by a self-interested pragmatism and blind to poverty and collective needs. Although Mrs Thatcher was voted into office in 1979 in part at least by an anti-Welfare State spending backlash, public support for such expenditure has grown in strength ever since – if selectively so, with strong support for the NHS, retirement pensions and education, as against benefits for the unemployed, single parents and children.[6] Moreover, public expenditure on Welfare State programmes has continued to increase throughout the period.[7] In interpreting such trends, two qualifications must be made. First, there is a growing geographical divide in attitudes, as in voting patterns. In the North and Scotland, a majority of the people believe in redistributing income to the less well-off and in increasing unemployment benefits (and vote Labour); in the economically more buoyant South, the proportions (and voting patterns) are reversed.[8] Interestingly, for the purposes of this chapter, the same pattern is evident in the proportion of the population taking out private health insurance: in the North and Scotland fewer people have such coverage than would be expected after allowing for the composition of the population.[9] Second, there is some survey evidence that 'private welfare is seen as superior to state welfare on almost every count' but that support for privatisation co-exists with 'countervailing sentiments of collectivism'.[10] Overall, then, the picture that emerges is an untidy one, with cross-cutting currents, that suggests an unwillingness either to abandon traditional collective responsibilities or to embrace the new consumerism without reservation: precisely what might be expected, in a period of transition and consequent intellectual turmoil.

We do not know to what extent public attitudes are shaped by Government policies, as distinct from Government policies being a response to voter preferences. But it is clear that the Thatcher Government has been committed to the principle that the market knows best, even though its practice has been more fitful and less consistent that its theory.[11] If the NHS was born in a period of nationalisation, it celebrated its 40th birthday at a time when the industries which had been taken into State-ownership in the 1940s were being sold off – with the pace quickening as the 1980s progressed. More generally, the pace of change picked up in the 1980s faster than might have been anticipated from the record of the first Thatcher Government – i.e. the period covered in Chapter 4 – and, in significant respects, changed emphasis if not direction.

In particular, it became clear that the Thatcher Administration's faith in market principles could not be equated (as had at first seemed possible) with less government. If the scope of government was reduced in some aspects, as by privatisation, its tread became heavier. In a sense, the Conservative Government can be seen as the equivalent of the Tudor Monarchy[12] asserting the power of the State in order to modernise a country previously dominated by feudal barons and corporate interests like the Church. To disperse the corporate groups that had created the sclerotic post-war consensus in support of their own interests (as the Tory revivalists saw it), the State had to use its authority to break them. It therefore needed more power, not less, if the corporate stalemate was to be broken and if Britain was to modernise its economy. In the first Thatcher Administration, the trade unions were tackled and tamed. Next, the second Thatcher Administration turned its attention to the quasi-professions and demonstrated the impotence of university and school teachers to resist government policies designed to reshape the education system. Finally, there are hints that even the most redoubtable professions – like lawyers and (as we shall see) doctors – will be forced to defend their claims to decide on their own restrictive practices in the name of autonomy. In short, the implicit vision of society is that of a strong, centralised State and strong, individualistic consumers – but with the role of intermediary bodies, be they local authorities, trade unions or professional associations, sharply diminished. In the case of education, for example, it is the State which has reduced the autonomy of both teachers and local education authorities in order to increase, so it is argued, the system's responsiveness to consumers.

The other continuing and developing trend has been the rise of the good housekeeping State. If the Government preaches and encourages self-reliance and the diffusion of responsibility, it is also intent on achieving efficiency. And, again, the paradox is that in order to achieve this policy aim, it must often forge new instruments of intervention. In pursuit of its value for money goals, it has adopted many of the techniques first developed in the 1960s and early 1970s by the rationalist managers (see Chap. 3, pages 64–65). Consider, in particular, the Financial Management Initiative (FMI)[13] which helped to transform administrative style throughout Whitehall and beyond – reaching even to the universities. The FMI philosophy is that each government programme should have explicitly stated objectives and measures of performance from which it is possible to assess progress towards the goals that have been set. So, for example, the annual Public Expenditure White Paper now sets out a series of objectives and targets for each spending programme, including the NHS. All this is not so very different from the notion of accountable units of management first put forward by the 1968 Fulton Committee on the Civil Service[14] or the contemporaneous advocacy of such techniques as programme budgeting. The real difference lies in the fact that, 20 years later, a very different kind of Government – preoccupied with a concern to contain public spending – has used this approach to create a new Whitehall management culture. In addition, of course, the technology for mobilising the information required for this kind of analytic approach has since become much cheaper, and therefore more widely available. Overall, however, the effect is to demonstrate the secularising or demystifying effect of using money to set a new agenda of questions about the purpose of government programmes: a ferret down the bureaucratic warren.

In pursuing a policy of centralising control over decision-making while decentralising activity, the Government was following some larger trends in society – and, especially, in the organisation of manufacturing, retailing and servicing industries. The trend is well caught in the following quotation from an industrialist, Sir Adrian Cadbury[15]:

> We will want, in future, to break these organisations down into their separate business units and to give those units freedom to compete in their particular markets. Large companies will become more like federations of small enterprises – not because 'small is beautiful' but because big is expensive and inflexible. ... I would expect tomorrow's companies ... to concentrate on the core activities of their business, relying for everything else on specialised suppliers who would compete for their custom.

In short, the trend is from centralised institutions to networks, from hierarchic, top-down models of organisation to looser constellations.[16] This fragmentation of traditional hierarchic models may not only have been made possible by developments in information technology but may also have been accelerated by them: given the rapid diffusion of knowledge, and given also the rapid pace of change, an adaptable peripheral learning model may be more appropriate and functional than a rigid central command model.[17] And what goes for the private sector applies, if anything with greater force, to the public sector. Thus it has been argued that: 'In a more complex environment top-down control becomes ineffective: instead the State becomes an overseer, a regulator of independent and competing organisations'.[18]

Such, then, are the main elements of the transformation of the environment in which the NHS operates. They were already evident in 1983 but awareness of their full logic has been slower in coming. The puzzle addressed in the rest of this Chapter is therefore not just how and why the NHS has changed but also how far and why the NHS has been insulated from the environmental pressures which have engulfed other institutions. Why, in short, has the NHS survived? Unless we assume that by some miracle the 1948 NHS provided the model of a perfect health service – and the whole argument of this book has been that, whatever the balance of its strengths and weaknesses, it was as much the product of messy compromises as of inspired visions – then this, surely, is the interesting question, rather than seeing any change or modification as an ideological onslaught on a sacred institutional inheritance and dismissing it accordingly.

PATTERNS OF CHANGE

In broad terms, four themes emerge from the history of the NHS since 1983. First, contrary to the trend of the early 1980s, but in line with the more general drift of government policy, there was a sharp turn towards centralisation. Far from decentralising responsibility and thereby diffusing blame, the Department of Health and Social Security moved towards setting objectives and monitoring progress towards their achievement. Second, and linked to this, there was a revival of faith in managerialism and bureaucratic rationality, again marking a change of emphasis from the start of the 1980s and a return (albeit unacknowledged and with variations) to many of the ideas fashionable in the 1960s and early 1970s. Third, there was a continuing, if unspectacular, expansion in the private sector and in the contracting out of services from the NHS, in line with the initiatives taken in the early 1980s. Fourth, there was a growing emphasis on the development of primary health care and prevention, as part of a wider strategy designed to stress the role of the consumer in exercising choice and responsibility.

In what follows, we shall examine each of these four areas in turn. What needs noting at this point is the apparent lack of consistency in the pattern revealed if one starts with the expectation that political ideology will determine policy outputs (see Table 1,

page 185). If some of the trends are very much in line with
the Thatcher Government's ideology, notably the rhetoric of
consumerism and private provision, these also tend to be the
policies where the overall impact of policy has so far been marginal.
Conversely, the policies which have been pursued most energetically
– the new emphasis on central direction and managerialism – would
almost suggest a reversion to a tradition of planning strongly
repudiated by the present Administration. In short, there would
appear to be as much evidence of pragmatism as of ideology, of
expediency as of design. There has certainly been a general drift
to 'welfare pluralism', as well as a new emphasis on a consumer-led
service as against a profession-led health care system.[19] But this
has been more significant in terms of the effect in changing
perceptions, and the agenda and rhetoric of political debate, than
in altering the structure of the NHS.

There is, however, one common element in the various themes
of government policy. They can all be seen as responses to the
central problem that has haunted the NHS since 1948: money.
The years following 1983 have been dominated by an increasingly
acrimonious political debate about the 'under-funding' of the NHS
(see below: page 229). And the whole battery of governmental
policy responses can be seen as the improvisations of an
Administration committed to conflicting policy objectives: to
cutting public expenditure while yet maintaining the NHS and
expanding its provision. No wonder, that – contrary to the analysis
and predictions of the previous chapter – the Government picked
out any and every available policy tool rather than selecting them
on ideological principles. The attempt to combine parsimony in
spending with adequacy of provision inevitably led Ministers to
seize on whatever instruments or devices happened to be at hand.
The question of money therefore not only links the various
themes running through this Chapter but also provides its grand
climacteric. There was a gradual escalation of the political debate
about funding until, as we shall see, the explosion of discontent
in 1987–88 that forced the Government to set up its Review of
the NHS: a Review which, ironically however, was to reaffirm the
Government's commitment to the organisational and financial
structure of the NHS. The last act of the play – when expectations
had been aroused that a combination of rising political embarrass-
ment and financial demands would bring about a fundamental
re-appraisal of the NHS – saw impending melodrama turn into
familiar farce: the corpse got up, and took its bow.

201

The politics of the National Health Service

In trying to make sense of this pattern of events and their outcome, a decisive factor – as we shall see – has been the balance between the political and financial costs to the Government. For the policy dilemma posed by the NHS for this, or any other, Government can be put in the form of a simple equation. On one side, are the demands generated both by NHS providers and consumers: the two, as argued previously, can in practice be separated only with difficulty since it is the former who largely shape the latter's expectations. On the other side of the equation, are the financial costs. To the extent that priority is given to satisfying demands, so the financial costs are likely to rise. To the extent that the financial commitments are contained, so the political costs of the NHS are likely to rise. The history of the post-1983 years can thus be seen as a succession of attempts to wriggle out of this dilemma – by introducing stricter central control and more effective management in order to wring more outputs out of any given volume of resources and encouraging demand to spill over into the private sector – which culminated in a Government decision to buy off the opposition by providing more funds for the NHS rather than to change the financial basis of the health care system. In effect, the Government concluded that even a slightly more expensive NHS (and a source of continuing, chronic political friction) was still preferable to any alternative, because cheaper and more effective.

This outcome is all the more in need of explanation because of the changes in the health policy arena that have been taking place. In contrast to the previous period, when the arena itself was expanding and new actors were taking their place on stage, the mid-1980s saw a contraction of the dramatic cast, or at least the relegation of some of the leading actors to walk-on parts. In line with what might have been expected from changes in the NHS's environment, the trade unions lost most of their ability to influence events: as we shall see, they failed in their opposition to the Government's contracting out and privatisation policies. In line with what might have been expected from the Government's hostility to all corporate groups, the overall aim of public policy was to enhance managerial influence at the expense of the medical profession: as we shall see, again, a series of decisions put a large question mark against the profession's continuing ability to veto change and to claim immunity from scrutiny in the name of autonomy. Finally, in line with the Government's determined push to assert central control, health authorities themselves increasingly came to be seen as agents of the Department of Health and Social Security rather than as representatives of the local community: a reversion to the 1948 model. In short, there was evidence that the protagonists of the politics of stalemate of the 1970s were beginning to lose their grip by the mid 1980s. Yet when it came to the point, a coalition of providers and the public persuaded the Government to retreat. The concentrated lobby of the former managed to mobilise the diffuse support of the latter.[20]

In noting the ability of the NHS providers to mobilise the public – specifically in convincing the public that more money should be spent – it is important to note also the growing salience throughout the 1980s of health care as a public policy issue. The two are linked, of course. For one reason for the growing salience of health care lies precisely in the fact that, as noted by Enoch Powell twenty years before (see Chap. 2, pages 54–55) the NHS providers have a vested interest in denigrating it: i.e. to advertise their own claims for extra resources by drawing attention to the shortcomings of the NHS. Hence the recurring 'crises' that have punctuated the history of the NHS, with prophecies of impending collapse surfacing roughly every three years. But the other reason lies in the increasing exploitation of health care as a political issue by all the opposition parties in the 1980s. In the 1983, and even more in the 1987, General Elections, health care turned into a major issue. So, for example, in 1987 'every poll showed that the NHS was Labour's strongest, and the Conservatives' weakest issue',[21] and all this despite the fact that more voters were taking the exit route into the private sector. Herein lies a paradox. On the one hand, the NHS has become politically more controversial than ever before. On the other hand, all parties embraced the NHS: the 1987 party manifestos competed in their hand-on-heart declarations of support for its principles.[22] So there is certainly more conflict than ever before, yet it still appears to be contained within consensus. But it is a consensus which may be more apparent than real since it contains disagreement about what the 'principles' of the NHS actually entail. It is as though rival religious sects were to lay claim to the body of the same saint in the name of their competing faiths.

What is most striking about all this, perhaps, is precisely the fact that the NHS still remains capable of inspiring so much quasi-religious passion. In this respect, little seems to have changed since the great battle over private practice in the 1970s (see Chap. 4). In the sections that follow, which examine specific areas, it is therefore important to remember that events and policies have to be interpreted as much in terms of their symbolic significance as of their practical implications.

THE RETURN TO CENTRALISATION

The policy of diffusing blame and disavowing government responsibility for what was happening at the periphery, as translated into the rhetoric of the 1982 reorganisation described in Chapter 4, was to have a short shelf-life. No sooner had Patrick (subsequently Lord) Jenkin implemented the reorganisation than he was replaced, as Secretary of State for Social Services, by Norman Fowler, who was to remain in office until 1987. While Jenkin was described by one of his own civil servants as too good a bureaucrat to be an effective Minister, Fowler was a supple, entrepreneurial politician. The style of the Department quickly changed. From repudiating the language of norm setting, and insisting that health authorities must have freedom to make their own decisions within broad national guidelines, the DHSS moved towards a system of performance review designed to monitor progress towards the achievement of very specific targets: a tighter system of control and accountability than had ever existed in the previous history of the NHS.

The switch reflected, of course, the general emphasis of Government policy as enunciated in the Financial Management Inititative. If the DHSS was to have any credibility with the Treasury in the annual battle for funds, it had to show that it was taking the FMI seriously. Additionally, a number of factors specific to the NHS, and springing from the very nature of the 1948 settlement, were prodding the DHSS in the same direction. For while the NHS remains overwhelmingly tax-financed, it is accountable to Parliament for the money spent: to return to one of the main themes running through the whole history of the NHS. And from 1980 to 1982 the DHSS was the target of a series of reports, from the Social Services and Public Accounts Committees of the House of Commons,[23] which cruelly documented and scathingly criticised its failure to find out what was happening at the periphery. At the same time the increasing emphasis on squeezing more value for money out of any given budget, reflecting not only the Government's over-optimistic commitment to reducing public spending but also the economic crisis of the early 1980s, put ever more pressure on the DHSS to intervene directly in the affairs of health authorities in order to ensure that its policies were being carried out.

The centre piece of the Department's new directive and interventionist strategy was the annual performance review, first launched in 1982.[24] Every year Ministers hold 'accountability meetings' with the Regional chairmen, where targets are agreed and progress towards them discussed. This is complemented by management meetings between the NHS Management Board (see next section) and Regional managers. The formal meetings are the 'culmination of the annual review process. This process is concerned with the identification and working up of the key issues for discussion and resolution'.[25] The Regions, in turn, carry out a similar exercise with each of their districts; finally district health authorities are expected to do the same with all their own sub-units. In short, there is a hierarchy of review and accountability running from the individual hospital to the Secretary of State.

Organisational innovation was supplemented by technical innovation: the introduction of a system of performance indicators.[26] Successive Ministers, almost from the birth of the NHS, had been frustrated by their inability to find out what was actually happening in the service. To the question of what was being delivered to whom, there were few and mainly unsatisfactory, answers. To the question of how to monitor, let alone assess, the changing performance of the NHS, there were even fewer, more unsatisfactory still, answers. In the 1970s, there was a brief flicker of interest in developing more adequate instruments, but this quickly waned as enthusiasm for the planning ideology of the 1974 reorganisation turned sour. As long as the emphasis of public policy was to set targets in terms of desired input of resources (so many beds, so many doctors, so many nurses per 1,000 population), adequate control could be exercised through the annual budget. But the growing preoccupation with value for money in the 1980s drew attention to the relationship between inputs and outputs. The focus of public policy switched to asking questions about *what* the money was buying. As Ministers faced hostile questioning from Parliamentary Committees about the adequacy (or otherwise) of NHS funding, so they increasingly switched to emphasising that improved productivity could yield more and better services even at a time of budgetary stringency.

The set of performance indicators (PI), first issued in 1983 and subsequently revised, can be seen in part at least as a response to such pressures. They were, and remain, an extremely crude set of instruments[27] using the available statistics routinely generated by the NHS. They were, and are, extremely vulnerable to questions about their accuracy and the time taken between collecting data and presenting it as PIs. They exclude many dimensions of performance, such as quality. But they do present, if in a rough and ready way, comparisons between the performances of different hospitals and different health authorities on a number of criteria, such as the cost per case treated, staffing levels related to patient numbers, waiting lists, the availability of particular services to any given population, and so on. As such they provide the policy makers and managers in the Department with tin-openers. They allow them to ask direct questions about what is happening at the periphery. A regional manager visiting the DHSS may be discomfitted to have some embarrassing aspect of his or her authority's performance flashed up on the VDU of the civil servant with whom he or she is speaking. In short, performance indicators have become a tool of the review system at all levels.

In all this, it is not just the revival of centralisation that is significant. It is centralisation speaking a different language, with the accent on outputs. If in the 1970s priorities were expressed in terms of inputs, by the mid 1980s they were being expressed in terms of targets of activity. Both points can be illustrated by taking the example of the 1985/86 round of regional reviews, and the outputs targets that emerged from them.[28] The Trent Region was set a target of 2,250 extra maternity patients, provoking somewhat ribald questions about who was to be responsible for increasing the birth rate; the West Midlands Region was set a target of 315 extra rheumatology patients, while the North Western Region was required to offer an additional 200 open heart operations and provide an extra 315 patients with renal dialysis treatment. Such targets are, of course, not arbitrarily imposed but are the product of negotiations between the DHSS and the regions: they represent figures which both sides believe to be attainable. But they are part of a new-style national strategy. Thus the annual Public Expenditure White Paper now publishes, in line with the FMI philosophy, national targets for the NHS as a whole. For instance, the 1988 White Paper[29] included the following acute sector targets to be achieved by 1990: an increase in the annual number of coronary artery by-pass grafts to 17,000 (from 10,500 in 1984); a rise in the number of hip replacement operations to 50,000 (from 38,000 in 1985) and an increase in the number of cataract operations to 70,000 (from 59,000 in 1985). Similarly, the DHSS set a national target for 40 new renal patients per million population to be accepted annually for treatment.

As these examples indicate, the objectives often tend to be a response to political pressures or worries. They are, in effect, a reply to criticism about the lengths of waiting lists (in the case of hip replacement surgery) or excessive harsh rationing (in the case of end stage renal treatment). In contrast to the 1974 reorganisation, where the emphasis was on central planning as the instrument of disinterested expertise, the 1980s brand of central interventionism was much more directly political, in the non-pejorative sense of being seen as the instrument for translating ministerial priorities into practice. It is precisely this which may help to explain why the new-style centralisation appears to have more vigour and life about it than its predecessors. The review system has been further reinforced as a transmission belt for the ministerial will by the gradual development, over the 1980s, of more direct contacts between politicians at the centre and district health authority chairmen at the periphery. Increasingly Ministers have brought their influence to bear directly on those responsible for carrying out their policies.

This 'politicisation' of the NHS can be interpreted in a variety of ways. From one perspective, it surely is right that Ministers should have the means of implementing the policies for which they (and no-one else) are accountable to Parliament. From another perspective, however, this is clearly at odds with the rhetoric of local accountability of the 1982 reorganisations of the NHS. In short, there may be a conflict between two different concepts of accountability which, as we have seen in previous chapters, have been at war with each other throughout the history of the NHS. And there is a further conflict. If the NHS is in any sense a 'democratic' institution (a dangerous because ambiguous term) it is precisely because it is politically responsive. In turn, to make a service as large and complex as the NHS responsive to Ministers means creating a managerial machinery capable of carrying out ministerial objectives. Yet the effectiveness of such a managerial machinery may depend on its ability to insulate itself from day-to-day political turbulence. In other words, there may be a trade-off between making the NHS so sensitive to day-to-day political objectives that it becomes incapable of pursuing even those longer term aims which Ministers themselves want to pursue. In the next section, therefore, we turn to the managerial revolution in the NHS.

THE NEW MANAGEMENT STYLE

In October 1983 there appeared a 25 page document which was to transform the management style of the NHS. This was the Report of the NHS Management Inquiry,[30] led by Sir Roy (as he subsequently became) Griffiths, managing director of one of the country's most successful supermarket chains, Sainsbury's. The style of the inquiry itself was to set the tone for its recommendations. It involved only four people. It took a mere six months to complete its tasks. It worked quickly and informally, consulting a great many people but not formally taking evidence. It thus marked a break with the tradition of setting up Committees and Royal Commissions, representative of all the interested parties, whose job it was to produce acceptable consensus reports: a break which has, more generally, been one of the hallmarks of the Thatcher Administration. The new management style in the NHS was thus born of an equally new approach to decision-making in Government – brisk and decisive, if sometimes also peremptory – and mirrored many of those characteristics.

The Griffiths Report's analysis was not new. In effect, it confirmed the diagnosis of institutionalised stalemate offered in Chapter 4. But it was expressed in blunt language. The NHS was suffering from 'institutionalised stagnation'; health authorities were being 'swamped with directives without being given direction'; the NHS was an organisation in which it was 'extremely difficult to achieve change'; consensus decision-making led to 'long delays in the management process'. In short, the report concluded in a phrase that was to reverberate through the media and across the years, 'if Florence Nightingale were carrying her lamp through the corridors of the NHS today she would almost certainly be searching for the people in charge'.

From this diagnosis followed a clear prescription: a general management structure from the top to the bottom of the NHS – i.e. individuals, at all levels, responsible for making things happen. At the top, within the DHSS, there was to be a Supervisory Board to be chaired by the Secretary of State to set objectives, take strategic decisions and receive reports on performance; below that, still within the Department, there was to be a Management Board led by a Chief Executive, to carry out the policy objectives, provide leadership and control performance; lastly, and perhaps most importantly, there were then to be general managers responsible for the operations of the NHS at all levels – regions, districts and units. The general managers, the report suggested, might well be recruited from outside the NHS or the civil service, while their pay and terms of service should be linked to their performance.

The recommendations were carried out almost to the letter. Both a Supervisory and a Management Board were set up within the DHSS. The arrangement was to prove unstable. The division of responsibility between them appeared to be blurred in practice; a power struggle developed between the civil service hierarchy of the DHSS and the Management Board.[31] The first Chief Executive of the NHS – Mr Victor Paige who had been brought in from industry – resigned because of the ambiguity about his role caused by the difficulty of drawing a firm distinction between political and managerial roles within the DHSS. The Minister of State for Health took over the chairmanship of the Management Board, while the Supervisory Board effectively withered away[32] – only to be resurrected, under a new name, by the 1989 Review. The experience suggests that, given the financial basis of the NHS, management is inextricably political in the sense of involving the Ministers who are accountable to Parliament: the endeavour to separate policy and management functions appears to be a never-ending battle. This was precisely why the 1979 Royal Commission considered but rejected the idea of an independent health commission to provide 'the permanent and easily identifiable leadership which the service at present lacks'.[33]

Within the NHS, however, the general management revolution swept on. Everywhere, at every level, new managers were appointed: some brought in from industry, commerce and the armed services but primarily old-style administrators re-born as managers, with a sprinkling of nurses and doctors. The consensus teams born in 1974 effectively died ten years later, and with them the attempt to institutionalise producer syndicalism; predictably so given the Government's general suspicion of corporate interest groups. The mobilisation of consent for change, rather than the consolidation of consensus, became the new style.[34] In effect, the medical and nursing representatives on the management team lost their veto power; in particular nurse managers lost much of the power they had gained after 1974 in the post-Griffiths era. The change, as Griffiths himself stressed[35] did not imply that managers would or should behave like 'a nineteenth century iron master. ... who is going to dictate every minute of the life of the consultant'. Managers, he argued, must involve clinicians in the decision making process. However, the new managers had, in contrast to their predecessors, a direct self-interest in the promotion of change. Their salaries and contracts were linked to performance; if they did not deliver the goods, they risked not having their contracts renewed (as happened to some of them, in the outcome).

A revolution in management style did not mean an immediate transformation of the NHS. The effects have depended much on individual personalities and the local environment, and may take a further decade or so to work themselves through the system. But for many managers the effects were liberating. There is, as the following quotations from district general managers illustrate,[36] a new sense that change is actually possible, a readiness to challenge professionals and a willingness to take risks:

What made me want to get into general management was a porter I passed every day at the main hospital entrance. He always had a fag hanging out of his mouth, he was rude to everyone – he just grunted – and yet, as Chief Nursing Officer, I could do nothing about it – I tried but I failed. As general manager I can.

A lot of Health Authorities spent most of their time talking about administrative and financial issues – and we were one of those. ... One of the most significant changes in this Authority is the number of items that appear on the DHA agenda that relate to nursing specifically or to medicine specifically. ... Now, in fact, I ask the questions and demand the answers and dictate – if need be – what the timetables are. So it's not the 'I'll do that when I feel like it' sort of approach.

The new style management is not about bringing clinicians to heel. Instead, it is about making them grow up. It's about making them take responsibility for doing things which they know in their hearts are right. ... It's my responsibility to promote the environment where this sort of activity can take place, but it's the general manager responsible for a particular clinical area who has the task of discussing with the clinicians in that area what are reasonable standards for them to set.

It is difficult to disentangle the specific effects of the post-Griffiths management style from other developments during the 1980s. The new confidence of management may have also reflected the Government's general success in facing down the trade unions, reflected in less militancy in the NHS among the ancillary workers who had been so prominent in the 1970s. Similarly, the financial pressures within the NHS (see below) may have given management more leverage in that managers had their own shrouds to wave in response to those traditionally displayed by consultants: the prospect of financial death as opposed to patient deaths. Overall, though, the above quotations indicate not just an increase in confidence but also a greater willingness to take on the NHS providers: to reject the claim, whether of porters or nurses or consultants, that they were autonomous in their own sphere and accordingly immune from scrutiny.

The new style was potentially subversive, too, of the traditional position of consultants. It may be no accident that, in the years following, the issue of how to discipline consultants – and, if need be, dismiss them – came up more frequently and prominently;[37] in contrast to the 1970s, and the kind of fatalistic inertia revealed by the Normansfield Inquiry (see page 130) managers were increasingly willing to act against inadequate or recalcitrant consultants. Equally subversive, furthermore, was the whole notion of setting objectives and targets and the linked system of review and performance indicators discussed in the previous section. For the ultimate logic of such a system of review is to challenge the performance not just of a particular health authority or unit within it but also that of individual consultants. Consider the case of waiting lists, politically one of the most sensitive issues throughout the 1980s, as it had been for much of the NHS's previous history. In fact, it was so sensitive that the Government provided some ear-marked funds with the specific purpose of reducing the queue. If waiting lists in a particular district are long, it may be because resources are inadequate (for which the Government can be blamed). Or the reason may be found in the way in which any given bundle of resources is managed by the district (for which the health authority can be blamed). Or it may be simply because of the work practices of individual consultants. For example, a study by John Yates[38] found the number of cases treated by individual orthopaedic surgeons varied five-fold, from 200 to 1,000 a year. Similarly, his analysis suggested that waiting lists reflected not so much a shortage of operating theatres but their under-use, an analysis subsequently confirmed by the National Audit Office (NAO).[39] And if it is the work practices of individual consultants which are responsible for long waiting lists – or, perhaps, above-average costs per case as revealed by the performance indicators – then, clearly, it is the job of an effective manager to challenge those practices: to invade, as it were, the sacred garden of professional discretion.[40]

Moreover, the traditional rights of consultants to determine which patients should be treated, and how, was being questioned from another perspective as well. Throughout the 1980s there was a rising interest in techniques designed to measure the relative impact of different medical procedures in terms of the cost of achieving specific outcomes. So, for example, one study compared the quality-adjusted life years (QALYs) yielded by heart transplants as against by-pass surgery.[41] Rising interest did not lead to consensus about the techniques; there was sharp disagreement about their validity and usefulness. But, potentially at least, it seemed that the technicians – economists, epidemiologists and others – might be able to provide managers with tools for determining medical priorities: a threatening prospect for consultants.

It would be misleading to imply, in all this, that the post-Griffiths era produced a direct confrontation between managers and clinicians. One theme of the Griffiths Report was precisely the need to engage clinicians in management and one of the main efforts of the NHS Management Board has gone into developing financial systems which would allow doctors themselves to manage their own budgets: yet one more example of how many of the ideas implemented in the 1980s represent the resurrection of notions first floated in the 1970s or even earlier,[42] rather than the importation and imposition of practices drawn from the world of supermarkets. The process has been more subtle and indirect than a direct challenge or confrontation. In a sense, the threat of managerial scrutiny may have been more important than its reality, to the extent that it persuaded the medical profession itself to examine, if only defensively, its own practices: again giving new life and new impetus to a debate which had started in the 1960s (see Chap. 3).

The trend towards critical professional self-examination was accelerated by the Griffiths Report both directly and as the unintended by-product of subsequent changes. One of the central arguments of the Report was that the management task revolved around delivering a good product to the consumer: 'Businessmen have a keen sense of how well they are looking after their customers. Whether the NHS is meeting the needs of the patient, and the community, and can prove that it is doing so, is open to question.' Thus, Griffiths put the question of how to define and enforce standards on the managerial agenda: was the quality of the goods being produced by the NHS adequate? Furthermore, quite accidentally, the post-Griffiths reshuffle created a lobby for quality. Jobs had to be found for dispossessed nurse managers and many of them re-emerged in charge of quality assurance – a phrase imported from the United States which was to become one of the hurrah terms of the 1980s.

Other factors were also pushing the medical profession in the same direction, factors which reflected wider changes in the NHS's environment. In particular, patients in the NHS services were becoming more like consumers in the market place in one respect. Given dissatisfaction with the product, they were more likely to seek redress from the law.[43] The Medical Protection Society (MPS) reported an increase in the number of claims of medical negligence received from 1,000 in 1983 to over 2,000 in 1987; the Medical Defence Union (MDU), the other major provider of insurance for doctors, reported a similar trend. At the same time the courts considerably increased the size of the awards made. The result was a sharp increase in defence society subscription rates: from £95 a year in 1980 to £1,080 in 1988. If Britain was still a long way from an American-scale 'malpractice crisis', the country seemed to be travelling in the same direction. No wonder, then that there was also growing interest in the medical profession in American-style quality assurance programmes designed to make sure that the product met required standards.

It is not clear, as yet, how far this interest in quality has prompted changes in practice as distinct from debate about future policy options. There has certainly been much of the latter. So, for example, it has been proposed that the Health Advisory Service (HAS) might become the model for a NHS inspectorate, though its own record hardly suggests that it has such a capability.[44] Similarly it has prompted interest in using hospital death rates as an indicator of quality – or rather as a negative indicator of things going wrong.[45] The medical profession has collaborated in a national study of post-operative deaths,[46] on the 20 year old model of the inquiry into maternal deaths, examining their possible causes – including medical mistakes. Finally, and perhaps most significantly, the Royal College of Physicians has decided that hospitals where doctors do not collectively audit their own work may lose their right to offer training posts to junior doctors.[47]

In all this, there is an irony. This is that much of the impetus for the increased emphasis on standards came from a report which explicitly took private, for-profit management as its model. In a sense, the NHS – which since its birth has been dominated by the belief that its 'publicness', its immunity from the corrupting effect of profit seeking, would guarantee high quality to the customer – has been forced to re-assess this assumption, and to recognise, if only implicitly, that it is a myth. It is a process which has been further accelerated by the growth of the private sector, to which we next turn.

A DRIFT TO PRIVATISATION

So far the analysis has tended to identify change rather than continuity in the 1980s, or at least new strategies for trying to deal with familiar problems. But there was one issue where little appears to have changed since the 1970s and where old political battles continued to be fought, testimony perhaps to the longevity of totems in politics. The word 'privatisation' still provoked the traditional reactions. In its 1983 manifesto the Labour Party pledged itself to 'remove private practice from the NHS and take into the NHS those parts of the profit-making private sector which can be put to good use'; in 1987, it took the view that 'privatisation means a Health Service run for profit rather than in the patients' interests. Labour will end privatisation in the NHS, relieve the pressure on NHS facilities by beginning to phase out pay beds and remove public subsidies to private health'. Conversely, the 1983 Conservative Manifesto, welcomed the growth in private health insurance and promised to 'promote' close partnership between the State and the private sectors in the exchange of facilities and of ideas 'in the interests of all patients'; in 1987, however, the emphasis switched to developments within the NHS itself. But 'privatisation' is a more complex concept than political stereotypes would suggest. It has a number of different meanings. On the one hand, it covers the private production of privately financed health care; the private sector in the strict sense. On the other hand, it is conventionally if inaccurately also used to describe the public purchase of services from the private sector: for example, contracting out laundry or catering services. Additionally, it may be used to describe one of the major developments of the 1980s, the provision of public funds to allow people to buy their own services in the private sector. Lastly, it has even been employed to describe the private financing of public services, ie. charges. In what follows, we shall therefore distinguish sharply between these various definitions, since each raises a somewhat different set of issues.

Throughout the 1980s, both the provision of acute medical care in the private sector and the proportion of the population with insurance policies continued to grow.[48] In 1979, there were 149 private hospitals with 6,600 beds; by 1988 there were 203 hospitals with 10,370 beds: an increase of more than 50 per cent in capacity.[49] In 1979, only 5 per cent of the population were covered by private health insurance schemes, by 1987 the proportion was edging towards 10 per cent.[50] It was not a consistent trend; a sharp rise in the early 1980s was followed by a sag in the middle of the decade. Significantly, it was a trend largely independent of Government policies. Despite manifesto rhetoric, the Thatcher Administration did nothing directly to encourage the growth of the private sector apart from increasing marginally (to a mere £8,500) the income limit below which tax concessions could be claimed for health insurance policies.

If, as argued in Chapter 5, private sector activity can be interpreted as a commentary on the failure of the NHS to respond to consumer demands, then its continued expansion growth would suggest a widening gap between what the public sector supplies and what the customers want. And this indeed was the interpretation put upon its growth by many of the Government's critics, who argued that the Government had starved the NHS of funds in order to drive demand into the private sector: that there was a deliberate move, therefore, towards creating a two-tier health care system. It is an argument which, however, needs to be unpackaged, since it conflates a number of different propositions.

First, there is little evidence of any change in the nature of the demand for private health care. It is still, overwhelmingly, for elective repair surgery for those conditions where there are waiting lists. It is for treatment to improve the quality of life for people of working age rather than to cope with life threatening conditions in the population as a whole. In all, an estimated 16.7 per cent of all non-abortion elective surgery in England and Wales was carried out in the private sector in 1986, with the proportion rising to over 28 per cent in the case of hip replacements.[51] Second, the evidence suggests that the growth of the private sector reflects not just frustrated access but also a demand for consumer-control over the timing of an operation, over who does the operation and over the physical environment.[52] The semantic transformation of passive patients (people to whom things are done) into active consumers (people searching out what the market offers) reflects the fact that, increasingly, men and women want to choose the timing of their treatment and the consultant who is to carry out the operation – goods not on offer in the NHS. Third, and following on from this, we could expect an increase in such demands simply because of the social and economic changes in the population noted at the beginning of this chapter. What we may be witnessing therefore is not increasing dissatisfaction with the NHS but a growing capacity to do what the wealthiest have always been able to do, which is to exit into the private sector when it suits them. There has always been a second tier but (like holidays abroad) it was until fairly recently reserved for a small minority. Fourth, and confirming such an interpretation, is the fact that demand for private health does not appear to be linked geographically to provision in the NHS. It is highest in the best-provided parts of the country ie. the London regions, and thus would appear to be linked to the characteristics of the population rather than to those of the NHS. Fifth, and crucially, the use of the private sector does not necessarily imply general dissatisfaction with the NHS. It represents, rather, a decision to shop around for a specific service in particular circumstances. Among those with private insurance coverage more than half the inpatient stays and four-fifths of the outpatient attendances were made under the NHS.[53]

Lastly, consumer demand in all health care systems is strongly influenced by medical decisions. Hence, the growth of the private sector may – if only at the edges – reflect incentives to doctors rather than patients. If anyone has done well out of the growth of the private sector, it is the medical profession. Private hospitals have suffered from under-occupancy – in 1987 the occupancy level was down to 55 per cent – and profits have at times been hard to make. The insurance companies have become increasingly preoccupied with cost-containment as expenditure and subscription rates have soared: BUPA's basic subscription rate for a family rose by 186 per cent between 1980 and 1987 compared to a 52 per cent rise in the retail price index.[54] But the medical profession's earnings have soared. In 1979 the insurance companies paid out under £37 million in medical fees; by 1987, this figure had topped £200 million. If these earnings were evenly spread across the consultant body, then it would imply an average income from private practice of almost £17,000 a year.[55] In fact, the distribution is skewed, and no doubt quite a few surgeons manage to double their basic NHS salaries, while geriatricians and others may earn well below the average.

Overall, it is therefore not surprising that the growth of the private acute sector has not eroded political support for the NHS. As noted at the start of this chapter this continued to be rock solid throughout the 1980s. The consumers do not exit into the private sector; they commute between it and the NHS. As a result neither voice nor loyalty is weakened. The medical providers handsomely benefit from a dual system. Strangely, the Review Body does not appear to take income from private practice into account when making its annual salary adjudication so that its analyses consistently underestimate medical earnings. And the insurance industry itself benefits from the existence of the NHS, where more than half of the beds are filled with precisely those customers who are of least interest for private insurers: the high-risk elderly. It might even be argued that the NHS itself benefits. Partly this is because, as previously argued, the private sector provides a safety valve for excess demand. Partly, too, it is because of the 'demonstration effect' offered by the private sector of opportunities for flexibility stifled in the NHS itself. For example, the private sector has shown that it is possible to deliver routine health care safely in much smaller hospitals than previously assumed – that quality does not necessarily depend on having a critical mass of consultants supporting each other – and that consultants do not require a retinue of junior doctors in order to be able to ply their craft.[56] For, crucially, the private acute sector is not independent of the NHS: it is the same consultants who operate in private hospitals as in the NHS. Not only does the economic viability of the private sector depend, to a large extent, on this symbiotic relationship, but it is also this, which continues to set a limit to its expansion.

The private acute sector represents a model of health care where people either buy insurance policies to cover the cost of their medical treatment in the market place or pay cash for care as and when the need arises, with the former method of payment dominating. The private sector of long-term care, as it developed in the 1980s, represents a very different model: cash payments for care, financed either by the patients and their families or through the social security system, with no insurance element. The number of beds for the elderly in private and voluntary nursing homes doubled, while that of beds for the elderly in private and voluntary residential homes almost tripled.[57] In contrast to the acute sector, where independent providers account for only a small proportion of total health care, the private and voluntary sector had overtaken the public sector as the largest producer of institutional long-stay care for the elderly by 1987. In what follows, the emphasis is on analysing the implications of the total growth in private provision, rather than distinguishing between the increase in nursing homes (roughly complementary to NHS services) and that in residential homes (roughly equivalent to local authority provision). In part, this is because functionally it is often difficult to separate nursing and residential homes; in part, it is also because the growth of both largely reflects a set of common circumstances.

For the boom in private institutional care for the elderly provides a case study of the dangers of looking for the causes of change exclusively in the dynamics of the health care policy arena or in the ideology of the government of the day. The health care policy arena could, perhaps, be better conceptualised as a large modern opera house with a revolving stage, where a new set of actors playing on a new set can be revealed by pressing a switch. In the case of institutional care for the elderly, for example, some of the leading actors found in acute medical care are missing. Consultants have little, if any, stake in the growth of this form of private provision; similarly this is a service industry dominated by small providers, usually owner-managers. This contrasts with the acute sector which is a capital intensive, relatively high-technology industry where large chains are prominent.[58] So the stage picture is very different, although the outcome appears to be the same. Nor does political ideology provide the explanation, even though the growth of the private sector fits snugly into the Government's preferences and has been fuelled by a large injection of public funds through the social security system.

But it is an injection of public funds which reflects not deliberate Government policy but the perverse and unintended effects of a series of decisions taken with quite different aims in mind.[59] Under the 1948 National Assistance Act, social security offices always had discretion to make allowances to those living in residential and nursing homes. From the 1970s onwards these payments slowly began to rise: by 1983 they had reached £39 million a year. The Department decided to stop the spending creep. Each social security office was asked to set limits for the weekly payments, reflecting the highest reasonable charge for the area. The result was precisely the opposite of that intended. The maxima quickly became the minima. More important, what had previously been a low-visibility discretionary payment overnight turned into a highly visible, as-of-right entitlement. The only test of need, in line with other benefits, was lack of financial resources to pay the required charges. The result, not surprisingly, was a sharp rise both in the number of residents whose fees were being paid by social security and in the level of charges. The spending creep turned into an expenditure avalanche. By 1986 social security spending on institutional care for the elderly had reached £500 million; by 1988

it was approaching, and may have exceeded, a billion. Contrary to
its policy aim of containing public expenditure, the Government
had created a demand-led, and therefore uncontrollable, spending
explosion. Contrary to its declared policy of targeting spending on
the most needy, the Government had created a new entitlement
where there was, in fact, no test of need for residential or nursing
home care. Consequently it generated perverse incentives to health
and local authorities to exploit social security's bias towards
institutional care, instead of developing community care.[60] Contrary
to its general ideological stance, the Government had furthermore
stumbled into the most egalitarian policy commitment taken during
its entire period in office. In effect, the social security entitlement
meant that the poorest had access to a service which previously
had been reserved for the relatively wealthy. So, in contrast to the
expansion of the independent acute sector, the growth of the private
and voluntary sector of institutional care has almost certainly
diminished rather than accentuated inequalities: a warning against
assuming that all the effects of 'privatisation' can be in one
direction only. If any lingering doubts remain about this being an
accidental and unintended policy outcome. it should be resolved
by the fact that the Government has anxiously sought to escape
from its commitment and to cap the social security expenditure:
a series of committees have reported,[61] and the only doubt that
remains is how the retreat is to be managed.

So the growth of private long-stay care for the elderly, and the
relative decline of the public sector, points to no simple ideological
moral. It does, however, raise two other general issues. First, it
emphasises the importance of environmental factors in explaining
what happens within the health care policy arena. Given the
increase in the over-75 population, demand for institutional care
might have been expected to rise irrespective of public policy.
Given the fact that an increasing proportion of the elderly were
becoming reasonably well off,[62] often with capital in the shape of
a house, demand for private institutional care might have been
expected to rise even if the public sector had been more generously
financed (and had not had an incentive to off-load demand onto
the social security system). As in the case of private acute hospitals
the geographical distribution of private institutional provision
reflects, among other factors, geographical variations in the social
composition of the population:[63] the wealthier the population, the
higher is private provision. Once again, then, social and economic
factors have to be invoked in trying to understand what is

The politics of the National Health Service

happening in the NHS. Second, the story is a further illustration of how developments in the private sector feed back into the public sector. In the case of institutional care for the elderly, the growth of the private sector provoked fears that vulnerable elderly people would be exploited by proprietors anxious only to maximise profits. The result was legislation in 1984 tightening up the responsibilities of health and local authorities for maintaining standards in nursing and residential homes: ie. for regulating the private sector.[64] But paradoxically the consequent debate about regulation raised, in turn, questions about the extent to which the NHS was maintaining standards for the vulnerable elderly in its care; hence adding to the pressure for improving quality noted earlier in this chapter. If exploitation for profit is frequently perceived to be the original sin of the private sector, exploitation of patients by providers is often revealed as the original sin of the public sector.[65]

The introduction of competitive tendering in 1983 would, at first sight, seem to provide a more clear-cut example of policy being shaped by the Government's new style and ideological stance. In September 1983 the DHSS issued a circular instructing all health authorities to put out to competitive tender their cleaning, catering and laundry services – which between them account for roughly 12 per cent of the NHS's total expenditure.[66] It was very much a central government directive specifying precisely the procedures to be followed, the criteria to be met and the time-table to be followed. Gone were the days when the DHSS merely offered guidance to health authorities, leaving them to interpret it in their own way and to proceed at their own pace; instead the Department took a detailed and intense interest in the process of implementation, frequently intervening directly and applying pressure to individual authorities. In its execution the introduction of contracting out thus provides a neat case study of centralisation at work, with Ministers making it very clear that they were determined to push their policies through, whatever the resistance or scepticism among NHS staff and members.

In the outcome, there was both resistance and scepticism. In particular, the principle of competitive tendering was seen as a direct threat by the NHS unions, NUPE and COHSE, which had been the leading actors in the battles of the 1970s (discussed in Chap. 4). Moreover, it was intended as such: competitive tendering, in effect, challenged the virtual monopoly of the in-house providers of services. The fact that the Government successfully pushed its policy through, despite a national campaign

220

by the unions and local attempts to block the tendering process, therefore illustrates the effect of changes in the NHS's environment on the balance of power within it. Developments in the NHS accurately reflected, in this respect, the general decline in the influence of the trade union movements. Similarly the Government's insistence on compliance with its policy directive on competitive tendering clearly underlined its determination that national policy objectives must override local preferences. Health authorities which appeared to favour in-house tenders from their own staff were sharply dealt with.

The direct financial yield of the new policy turned out to be relatively modest. By 1986 annual savings had reached £86 million.[67] Furthermore, the policy did not 'privatise' the NHS's support services in the sense of transferring them to the private sector. Of all the contracts awarded by the end of the first cycle of tendering in 1986, only 18 per cent went to private contractors. The rest were all awarded to bids coming from in-house teams, which by the end of the period were capturing over 90 per cent of all contracts. But if the direct effects were less than spectacular, the indirect effects were more significant. The exercise forced NHS managers to examine what they were doing. When it started most of them had never specified the standards of their services, let alone devised ways of defining quality of provision: for, although the exercise prompted many complaints about a consequent decline in quality, it was never clear on what these were based – since no previous benchmarks existed. In addition, apart from forcing improvements in the techniques of control, the contracting out process also gave confidence to managers. It demonstrated that change could be introduced and resistance could be overcome. Overall, then, the gains in efficiency may have been both larger and less visible than the figures of direct savings suggest. So, too, were the costs of the exercise which tended to fall on the lowest-paid and most vulnerable workers in the NHS. The price of successfully defending in-house services tended to be lower earnings and redundancies.[68] Overall, therefore, contracting out can be seen most accurately not so much as the product of an ideology of privatisation but as the product of an ideology of managerial efficiency. After all, it was a Labour Prime Minister – Harold (subsequently Lord) Wilson – who pioneered the concept of contracting out, when in 1968 he decreed that central government departments should find private contractors to take over their cleaning. The Conservative strategy is therefore best interpreted as an attempt not so much to transfer the production of health care to the for-profit sector as to introduce some of the disciplines of competition into the NHS.

The Government's enthusiasm for privatisation also turns out to have been heavily qualified when one examines, finally, yet another sense in which the word has been used. This is the process of 'privatising' health care costs by charging patients. For instance, it has been argued that the increase in various charges to patients under the Conservative Administration represents a 'backdoor privatisation' of services.[69] Leaving aside the question of whether or not this is an appropriate use of the term, some other qualifications need to be noted. The increases represent a policy of cautious incrementalism, rather than a sudden rush of ideological blood to the head. Conspicuously, the increases have fallen most heavily on precisely those services which, rightly or wrongly, have been perceived from the 1950s onward as most marginal to the main purposes of the NHS: dental and optical services. And in the sensitive area of prescription charges, there has been no attempt to widen the revenue base by narrowing the exempt categories. Conversely, of course, with 75 per cent of all those getting prescriptions in the exempt category, it means that any rise in charges falls entirely on the remaining quarter. Interestingly, too, private expenditure on over-the-counter remedies greatly exceeds spending on prescriptions. Most significantly, perhaps, the Government resisted the arguments for widening the scope of charges by extending it from primary care to the hospital sector. Not surprisingly, the total effect of this form of privatisation – if that is what it was – has been slight. In 1979/80 charges contributed 2.2 per cent. of the NHS's total finance; in 1987/88 the proportion was 2.8 per cent. – considerably less than it had been in the early 1970s, and very much less than it had been in the 1950s.[70] This is therefore an example of continuity in policy making, rather than marking a break with the past. If the position of patients is changing, it is not because they have to pay significantly more for medical care but because of their rhetorical transformation into consumers, as already noted. And the next section turns to analysing the implications of this in the case of primary care.

CONTROLLING THE GATEKEEPERS

One of the paradoxes of the NHS since its creation has been that it exercises least control over those who, in theory at least, exercise the greatest influence in determining the demand for health care: general practitioners.[71] It remains unique in the special role and status given to GPs. They are, at one and the same time, the patient's agents in steering him or her to the appropriate specialist and the system's gatekeepers in that they determine who is referred where and for what. But they are also independent contractors. In effect, they are small businessmen who – as noted in previous chapters – have fiercely and successfully defended this status ever since 1913. Despite changes in the small print of the GP's contract – especially those introduced by the Family Doctor Charter of the 1960s (discussed in Chap. 3) – general practice has in effect remained an autonomous enclave within the NHS: a fact recognised by the 1982 decision to make Family Practitioner Committees, the bodies responsible for the administration of primary health care, bodies independent of the NHS managerial structure and directly accountable to the DHSS. It was a decision which also reflected, as previously noted, the political costs of tangling with general practitioners; painful, ancestral memories of decades of wrangling with the BMA were slow to die in the DHSS.

But as the 1980s progressed, it became increasingly clear that the financial costs of avoiding a confrontation with the medical profession over general practice might outweigh any political costs. The emphasis on improved management might allow the NHS to cope with more demand within any given budget; the development of the private sector might provide a safety valve for excess demand. But none of these strategies could address the question of whether it was possible to limit the seemingly inexorable upwards surge of demand itself. Was it inevitable that, given the rise in the over-75 population and given the new possibilities of treatment opened up by technological change, demand would go on rising? Or was it possible to devise other strategies which might at least limit the rate of expansion?

As the questions became more urgent in the 1980s, so inevitably attention turned to primary health care and to prevention. Indeed, primary health care could, itself, be seen as a form of prevention: i.e. as a means of coping with conditions either before they became acute enough to call for more expensive hospital intervention or as a way of providing treatment more cheaply than in an institutional setting. In addition, primary health care was a source of obvious concern for a Government anxious to control public spending. It represented an open-ended public expenditure commitment; there was no way of imposing cash limits on the amount spent by GPs in prescribing, just as there appeared to be no way to check the number of people they referred to hospitals. There were wide, seemingly inexplicable variations in the rate at which different GPs prescribed and referred – a range of 20 to one – yet public policy seemed incapable of bringing discipline to apparent chaos. The number of GPs in practice increased; average list sizes fell below the 2,000 mark; the salary bill for helpers employed in surgeries shot up; yet, frustratingly, there was little evidence that the increased investment in general practice was yielding any returns. Neither prescribing nor referral patterns seemed to be linked systematically to such factors as list size.[72]

It was not surprising, then, that prescribing provided the first demonstration of the Government's willingness to risk political costs in order to bring financial costs under control. Not only did spending on prescribing account for almost half the total expenditure on primary health care; it was also expanding at a rate of more than 5 per cent. a year in real terms.[73] The notion of restricting the established right of general practitioners to prescribe whatever they wished, regardless of the cost of the drugs and the availability of cheaper substitutes, had been floating around a long time. Successive Governments had, however, flinched from the prospect of a head-on conflict with the BMA on this issue. Hence the announcement of a 'limited list', in November 1984, caught everyone by surprise.[74] It created what Norman Fowler, the Secretary of State, described as an 'eccentric alliance' in opposition to the proposal between the medical profession, the pharmaceutical industry and the Labour Party. The BMA, angered at the unprecedented failure of the government to consult the medical profession before taking a policy decision, protested strongly at what its Secretary described as 'one of the biggest changes in the NHS since its introduction'. But Kenneth Clarke – then Minister of State for Health – told them sharply that 'private formal consultation' in advance of publishing proposals was 'no way to run a system of parliamentary government': a remark which, like the confrontation itself, carried uncanny echoes of Nye Bevan's battle with the medical profession almost 40 years previously. The drug industry launched a major campaign against the proposal, on the grounds that it would introduce a two-tier system of medicine by discriminating against those patients who could not afford to buy drugs excluded from the official list and, predictably, that the resulting cut in profits would restrict research designed to produce new products. More surprisingly the Labour front-bench criticised the proposals as a 'major threat to the NHS' and echoed the drug industry's assertion that it would introduce the two-tier principle.

In the event, confrontation ended in compromise. Some of the Government's backbenchers were restive; the medical profession itself was divided, with support for the principle of the limited list from some of the Royal Colleges; the Opposition, too, was split. In February 1985 the Government announced that the limited list would be extended from 30 to 100 items and that the medical profession would be consulted about its precise composition; an Advisory Committee on NHS Drugs was set up to consider proposals for adding new drugs to the list; the estimate of likely savings was pared down from £100 to £75 million a year. But the Government had successfully imposed the principle of a limited list and, in so doing, provided further evidence that its willingness to take on corporate interest groups could extend even to the medical profession. It had challenged the idea that clinical autonomy bestows an automatic right to use public resources without scrutiny or limits. Lastly, it had once again demonstrated that, in its pursuit of efficiency, it was prepared to use any tools, whether or not consistent with its ideology of the market and minimum State interference: in this case, the tools of bureaucratic control.

The tension between managerial and market strategies, between bureaucratic control and consumer choice, also marked the Government's proposals for the reform of primary health care first unveiled in 1986. The Government's discussion document[75] set four main objectives. The first two were 'to give patients the widest range of choice in obtaining high quality primary health care services' and 'to encourage the providers of services to aim for the highest standards and to be responsive to the needs of the public': what might be called consumer-oriented objectives. The second pair were 'to provide the taxpayer with the best value for money from NHS expenditure' and 'to enable clearer priorities to be set for the family practitioner services in relation to the rest of the NHS': what might be called the managerial objectives.

The specific proposals reflected this mix of motives. On the one hand, there were a set of proposals designed to make GPs more sensitive to consumer preferences. This was to be done mainly by increasing the proportion of the doctor's income represented by capitation fees (which had sunk to 45 per cent. by the mid 1980s) and to make it easier for patients to change their doctors – so, in short, sharpening the incentives of GPs to satisfy their customers.

225

In addition, the discussion document put much emphasis on increasing the availability of information to prospective patients about the services provided, again reflecting the desire to create more of a market situation. On the other hand, there were a set of proposals designed to increase control over the activities of GPs and other contractors. This was to be done largely by strengthening Family Practitioner Committees (FPCs), hitherto viewed as managerial eunuchs whose chief responsibility was to shuffle papers and pay out money. Their responsibility was to be to carry out a 'regular appraisal of the quality and quantity of services being provided' and 'to develop more systematic means of measuring quality and detecting shortfalls in the provision of services'. Additionally, the 1986 document floated the idea that GPs themselves might be given a direct incentive to improve standards by being offered 'good practice allowance'. Entitlement might be contingent both on objective measures like 'personal availability to patients' and a performance review which might include 'such things as prescribing patterns and hospital referral rates'.

There followed, in this case, a highly visible exercise in consultations during which Ministers took evidence from 370 witnesses representing 73 organisations. In addition, the House of Commons Social Services Committee published its own inquiry.[76] If the intention was to increase the Government's freedom of manoeuvre by promoting a babble of conflicting voices, the strategy succeeded. The White Paper published in 1987[77] remained faithful both to the objectives and to most of the proposals put forward in the discussion document. There were some clear concessions to the medical profession. The idea of a good practice allowance was dropped. But there was greater emphasis, if anything, on strengthening the role of FPCs and establishing managerial control over general practice:

By ensuring that they receive more information about the services for which they are responsible and improving their means of control, the Government will require FPCs to exercise a stronger role in the management of those services. In this way the Government expects to secure continuing improvements in the level, quality and cost effectiveness of service provision and greater accountability.

Specifically, FPCs were to be given a new set of responsibilities. These included setting disease prevention targets, carrying out consumer surveys 'to ensure that the views of the public are obtained and taken into account' and monitoring, with the help of independent professional advice, the pattern of referrals to hospital.

The politics of modernisation

In all this, there was a conflict between the different objectives.[78] If consumer choices is to bite, there has to be competition for customers between providers. But if there is to be such competition, it is difficult to see the logic of maintaining the 1948 system that restricts the right of GPs to set up shop where they wish. This system was devised, as we saw, to ensure a better distribution of medical manpower but is difficult to justify in an era when the increasing availability of women doctors means that there is no longer a shortage of would-be general practitioners.[79] But any expansion in the number of GPs runs counter to the Government's objective of containing costs to the extent that each extra practitioner may swell the drugs bill and add to the numbers of referrals. Furthermore, it is not clear as yet how effective FPCs can be in establishing managerial control, since GPs firmly remain independent contractors.

The Government's 1987 White Paper also gave prominence to a new but fast developing theme in the evolution of its health policies. Its title *Promoting Better Health*, provides the clue. By 1987 the Thatcher Administration had become converted, with some enthusiasm, to the cause of health prevention. The White Paper added a new objective to those enunciated in the consultative document. This was 'to promote health and prevent illness'. It gave much more emphasis to the role of GPs, both in advising patients about life-style and in screening at-risk groups, particularly the elderly; moreover, it reinforced rhetoric with financial commitment by proposing to introduce appropriate payments as incentives. Indeed 'the prevention of avoidable illness and the promotion of good health' feature as the first of the six principles guiding Conservative policies on health care in the party's 1987 election manifesto, and the point was further elaborated in a long catalogue of initiatives: for example, a 'major campaign to tackle the problem of coronary disease'. The impact of the commitment is less significant – since it is too early to come to any conclusions on this point – than the fact that the Government chose to move in this direction at all. Health prevention and promotion in the past tended to be enthusiasms of the Left; thus in our analysis of likely policy response in Chapter 6 (Table 1, page 185) prevention was presented as the strategy most likely to be pursued by collectivists. Why did this prediction go wrong and what do the reasons for this mis-prophecy tell us about the politics of the NHS in the late 1980s?

In the first half of the 1980s, the Government showed little enthusiasm for prevention and promotion. It quarrelled with the Health Education Council and subsequently reformed it, in part at least because of the latter's obsession with the issues raised by the Black Report on social inequalities in health. There was a steady decline in the status and role of community physicians; the medical specialists who, in the 1974 reorganisation, had been cast in the role of the philosopher kings who would establish need and determine priorities according to their own, technical criteria.[80] But, then, came the conversion. It appears to have had two causes: AIDS and money. By 1986 the Government had become intensely worried about AIDS,[81] responding less perhaps to the number of deaths (which were still few) than to the number of column inches in the press (which were many). A Cabinet Committee was set up; a major House of Commons debate was held. But what characterised this new epidemic was precisely that it was not immediately amenable to laboratory science or medical treatment. The only policy instruments that appeared to be available were the traditional public health tools. In particular, the Government committed itself to a major campaign of public health education, given that the only long-term protection against the spread of AIDS appeared to be a change in the population's sexual habits. The epidemic thus created a new constituency of support for preventive strategies and strengthened the influence of Sir Donald Acheson, the Chief Medical Officer, within the Department: the main protagonist of the public health tradition as represented by community physicians. But the other reason which might explain the new-found enthusiasm was, as always, money. As suggested at the beginning of this section, if demand seems to be set on a collision course with supply, Governments will inevitably be drawn into searching for means to manipulate the former. The new emphasis on reducing demand by controlling GPs was one such policy response; the new stress on preventing illness was another, all the more so since it fitted neatly into the Conservative rhetoric about individual responsibility. In the next section we turn to the theme which has underlain all the policy variations discussed so far but which has yet to emerge explicitly and fortissimo: the financing of the NHS.

GÖTTERDÄMMERUNG – AND BACK AGAIN

One of the most tiresome aspects of Wagner's Ring is that, in each of the four operas which make up the cycle, the characters recapitulate everything that has gone before at tedious length. It is a narrative device designed to remind the audience that the whole action – including the final conflagration in the concluding opera, Götterdämmerung – springs from a crucial moral flaw in the opening one: when Wotan, the Head God, acquires a hoard of gold by deception. It is this which provides the dramatic logic of the whole cycle. In a sense, it is tempting to write the political history of the NHS in much the same way, starting with the fact that the Founding Minister, Nye Bevan, failed to endow the NHS with sufficient gold.[82] It is precisely because of this that, as we have seen throughout this book, any analysis or narrative has to keep on reverting to the built-in tensions that spring directly from the original failure to base the funding of the NHS on anything more solid than the shifting sands of political fashions and governmental preferences. And it would provide a neat dramatic climax to this book if, in this final chapter, the curtain could come down on the NHS in financial flames. Instead, as we shall see, there was to be no Götterdämmerung – but a final anticlimax as the firemen led by Kenneth Clarke, the Secretary of State, rushed onto the stage to douse the fire with buckets of money in the last Act.

It was a near-run thing. As the 1980s went on so the chronically recurring financial crisis of the NHS appeared to become ever more acute. By the beginning of 1988, when the Prime Minister announced a radical review, NHS underfunding seemed to be terminal. In discussing the reasons for this sense of doom, the obvious starting point is the level of spending itself. Compared to the 1970s, the 1980s were years of financial stringency. Over the entire period from 1980–81 to 1987–88, current spending on the hospital and community health services rose by only 10 per cent in real terms even including the funds internally generated by the Government's cost improvement drive.[83] It was a considerably slower rate of expansion that in the previous decade, although the decline in the annual increment had already begun in the second half of the 1970s as noted in Chapter 4. Even the technical question of how to calculate these figures – for example what figures to use for the rate of inflation in NHS prices and wages – produced considerable controversy. However, for the purpose of this analysis, a more relevant focus than the odd disputed percentage point is the debate about how to interpret the expenditure figures as it developed over the 1980s: the debate between the 'inputers' and the 'outputers', between the Government's critics and successive Secretaries of State.

The criticism of the Government's expenditure plans, as articulated by the all-party Social Services Committee of the House of Commons in a succession of reports, drew attention to a widening gap between the actual input of resources and what was required. To define what was required, the Committee used criteria first devised in the 1970s by the DHSS itself in order to extract money from the Treasury: an exercise in ingenuity by some anonymous civil servants which was to haunt their departmental colleagues in the 1980s. These produced an annual growth target of about 2 per cent. As one much quoted Ministerial statement[84] put it:

One per cent is needed to keep pace with the increasing number of elderly people: medical advance takes an additional 0.5 per cent and a further 0.5 per cent is needed to make progress towards meeting the Government's policy objectives (for example to improve renal services and develop community care).

Comparing actual spending levels with the expenditure needed to produce an annual growth of 2 per cent, it was then a simple arithmetical exercise to produce a figure of the total under-funding of the hospital and community services. Using this method, the Social Services Committee in 1986 produced a figure of £1.325 billion as the cummulative under-funding since the start of the decade. It was a figure which was to reverberate throughout the entire debate, feeding alike the sense of grievance within the NHS and the indignation of Opposition politicians. And when the Social Services Committee repeated its exercise in 1988, it came up with the still more dramatic figure of £1.896 billion as the accumulated deficit.

The Government, in contrast, put the emphasis on outputs, i.e. on what the NHS was actually producing. This, of course, was the logic of a value for money approach which inevitably hinges on the *relationship* between inputs and outputs and defines performance in terms not of the level of resources but of activity. Already in 1983, the Government's preparation for the General Election, included the publication of a document setting out the increase in activity, like the rise in the number of patients treated.[85] And this remained the Government's response to criticism throughout the 1980s. Thus in its evidence to the 1988 Social Services inquiry.[86] the DHSS provided figures showing the increase in the number of cases treated and in specific operations. For instance, hip replacement operations increased from 44,800 to 53,000 between 1980 and 1985, while heart operations rose from 27,200 to 43,000. Overall, the figures showed that rising productivity had indeed meant improving access – measured in terms of the rate of treatment by age bands – for the population as a whole, despite the persistence of waiting lists. But, then, the political salience of waiting lists has been in an inverse relationship to their actual significance throughout the history of the NHS, given the evidence that they are as much an artefact of individual clinical policies as a measure of frustrated demands. As presented by the Government, the statistics appeared to show that the NHS was a success story despite alleged financial shortfall.

The debate turned out to be a dialogue of the deaf. The Government's logic in directing attention to the outputs of the NHS was impeccable. The level of inputs tells us nothing of itself: any given bundle of resources can be either adequate or inadequate depending on the way it is used. However, the Government's line of reasoning was vulnerable on two counts. First, its story about increasing activity and improved productivity could say nothing about the adequacy of what was being produced. Given the lack of any measure of demand – let alone need – increasing activity could still be compatible with a shortfall in what was required. Second, it was argued that improved productivity – as reflected, for example, in shorter average lengths of stay by hospital patients – was being achieved by cutting quality and decanting problems into the community. Again, given the lack of any generally accepted measures and relevant evidence, it was a criticism which could not be proved or refuted. The demonstration of underfunding by the Social Services Committee was similarly flawed.[87] The precise figure of the under-funding depended crucially on the base-line chosen. Yet there was no particular logic about choosing 1980 as the starting point for the exercise; there is no way of telling whether the NHS was over or under funded in that year. So the deficit, as calculated by this method, could just as easily be twice as large or non-existent. Finally, the method extrapolates into the future costs based on past practices at a time when it is public policy to change those patterns of service delivery (and when the client populations concerned, particularly the elderly, are also changing: tomorrow's over 75s will be more prosperous, and perhaps also healthier, than today's.)

Nor do the problems of resolving the dispute between the 'inputers' and 'outputers' end there. To concentrate exclusively on expenditure on the hospital and community services – as the whole debate did – is to exclude a variety of highly relevant factors. On one side of the balance sheet, it excludes possible changes in the pattern of demand for health services caused by socio-economic factors, such as unemployment. On the other hand, it ignores other areas of rising public expenditure. So, for instance, none of the figures take into account the extra money channelled into long-stay care for the elderly through the social security system nor, more strangely still, the fast increasing expenditure on primary health care. Finally, no one – not even the Government – raised the question of whether or not the extra spending on private health care should be brought into the reckoning. If all these had been taken into account, it is quite possible that in 1988 there was no under-funding of health care in Britain (as distinct from, possibly, the NHS) on the basis of the Social Services Committee' own methodology. However, the 1980s debate was a dialogue of the deaf precisely because there was no agreement on the currency of argument and no consensus about how to define key terms like adequacy, need or quality. Lacking such an agreed vocabulary and generally accepted measuring rods, no resolution was possible. There was little the technicians – whether statisticians or epidemiologists, economists or social policy experts – could do to resolve the dispute. It was inevitably and inescapably politicised. And therein, precisely, lies the real significance of the debate. Its nature was defined less by the issues involved than by the characteristics of the policy arena.

Insofar as the characteristics of the policy arena had remained unchanged, so the 1980s debate over funding mirrored the disputes that had regularly punctuated the history of the NHS over the previous 30 years. The reason for its regular recurrence is, as argued throughout this book, built into the very structure of the NHS. If health service providers are to secure more resources for themselves, they can best advertise their case by pointing to the shortcomings of the NHS. What does need explaining about the 1980s – and in particular, the climactic confrontation between the medical and nursing professions and the Government in 1987 and 1988 – is the scale and ferocity of the conflict.[88] It was marked by a concerted and determined attempt by the providers to demonstrate that the NHS was on the point of collapse and thus to mobilise public opinion in a campaign for extra funding. The Presidents of the Royal Colleges warned the country of impending disaster; the President of the Institute of Health Service

Management called for a radical review of the NHS; the Committee of Vice Chancellors rumbled ominously about the threat of declining standards of medical education and research. Never before in the history of the NHS had there been such a public demonstration of concern, involving all the authoritative figures in the health care policy arena.

Moreover, these concerns were dramatised almost daily in the newspaper headlines and television programmes which translated abstract questions about finance into human terms. Again, both the extent and intensity of the coverage was unprecedented in the history of the NHS (how much this tells us about the NHS as distinct from the changing nature of the media is another matter, of course). There was a succession of reports about hospital wards which had to be closed because of cash shortages. There was a procession of consultants complaining about being unable to carry out life saving operations because of lack of resources. There was a rash of strikes by nurses in protest about closures and shortages. The BMA's Central Committee for Hospital Medical Services commissioned a survey to document the impact of financial inadequacy,[89] and came up with statistics of bed closures, cancelled operating sessions and staff shortages. The picture that emerged forcibly and vividly from all these accounts was that of a health service where the staff felt themselves to be unable to deliver care of adequate quality, where patients were being turned away and where morale and standards were both plunging. Given the obvious passion and conviction of those putting the case, it was difficult for Ministers to find a convincing response. Statistics about continuing rises in the number of patients treated and of operations carried out appeared unpersuasive in the face of so many witnesses testifying to decline and disintegration.

Moreover, if there was confusion about what was happening in the NHS, it was in large part because the evidence was extremely confusing and difficult to interpret. What was to be made of bed closures? The NHS had been reducing the number of acute beds throughout its history; beds are, in any case, a poor indicator of resource availability since what matters crucially is the intensity with which they are used and the supporting staff levels. As many beds were closed in 1977 and 1978 as in 1987 and 1988.[90] So what was different about the 1980s? One answer to this question only compounded the difficulties of providing a clear and simple picture. The 1980s were marked by increasing divergences between the experiences of different health authorities. This, paradoxically, was the perverse outcome of the 1970s RAWP formula (see Chap. 4, p 131) for equalising resource distribution between regions. Although the desired outcome was equality between health districts, the process of moving towards this objective inevitably meant *more* inequality in the annual allocation of funds: with more going to those districts judged to be below their appropriate funding level, and less going to those deemed to be relatively over-funded. A formula invented in a period of optimism about continued budgetary increases, and so designed to achieve a politically painless redistribution through differential growth rates, came to mean cuts for some districts in a period of fiscal stringency. While some health authorities were notching up an annual increase of 5 per cent, in real terms, others had their budgets reduced.[91] So the impression of cuts in the NHS was accurate enough but was inaccurately generalised to the service as a whole: hence the paradox of the rhetoric of cuts in a period of continuing, albeit very slow, growth. The fact of wide variations in the financial situation of individual health authorities – as well as in the nature of local problems and in the competence of local managers to handle them – tended to be overlooked amid the general hubbub.

The perception of a generalised crisis reflects two other factors special to the health policy arena of the 1980s. The first is technical. The system of cash-limits introduced in the late 1970s and consolidated in the 1980s meant that, at the start of each financial year, the Government allocated a sum of money to the NHS (as to its other programmes) with provision to cover any price or wage and salary rises. The rationale of this was to introduce financial discipline. If costs went up, then those responsible for the spending programme would have to absorb them within their cash limits. But Governments, anxious to discourage high pay claims, invariably under-estimated likely increases. Furthermore, in the case of the NHS, decisions over wage and salary increases are national, while responsibility for budgetary control is local. The result was to politicise the cash limits system. Every salary or wage award – whether to doctors or nurses or other NHS workers – was followed by a battle between health authorities and Government. The former invariably argued that the cash limits did not adequately cover the cost of the settlement: an argument rarely stilled even when the Government provided supplementary finance. In other words, the cash limits system reinforced the incentives of those working in the NHS, and in particular the managers, to advertise the inadequacies of their budgets.

The second factor sharpening perceptions of crisis in the 1980s was the managerial revolution, reviewed in the earlier parts of this chapter. In the case of nurses one effect was, as we have seen, to weaken their position in the managerial hierarchy. The post-Griffiths changes could thus be seen by them as an attack on the status to which they had aspired so long and which they had appeared to win in the 1974 reorganisation. In the case of the medical profession, the new managerialism presented a potential threat to their clinical autonomy as traditionally conceived; their immunity from scrutiny appeared to be at risk. In short the basis of the implicit concordat on which the NHS was founded – that Ministers would decide on resource levels while consultants would have complete autonomy within any given budget – seemed to be in the process of being eroded. No wonder, then, that disguising political decisions about resource allocation as professional decisions about clinical policy[92] was becoming less appealing, and that the case for explicit political rationing decisions was being argued more frequently.[93] No wonder, too, that the medical profession's sense of insecurity translated itself into low morale and a tendency to see the chronic shortcomings of the NHS as an acute crisis. If rationing by consultants had always been a fact of life in the NHS, it was perhaps becoming less attractive to accept responsibility for it during the second half of the 1980s and more tempting to blame the Government.

Whatever the causes of the campaign, the Government bent under the pressure. First, in January 1988, came the Prime Minister's announcement of a review of the NHS. Second, there followed a succession of extra top-up grants to finance pay awards. Third, in July Kenneth Clarke was appointed as the Secretary of State of a Department of Health, shorn of its social security functions. He succeeded John Moore who, in his year at the DHSS, had signally failed to cope with the storm. Fourth, in November, the new Secretary of State announced that in the annual public expenditure round he had managed to extract an extra £1.8 billion for the NHS for the coming financial year[94] – almost precisely the figure of 'under-funding' produced earlier in the year by the Social Services Committee. The message of this succession of events was clear and set the stage for the publication of the long-awaited Review: the Government had reaffirmed its commitment to the NHS and damped the excited speculation that its Review would lead to the creation of a new system of financing and organising health care in Britain.

CONFLICT RESOLVED OR POSTPONED?

The Prime Minister's announcement of a Review of the NHS in January 1988 precipitated an intense flurry of pamphleteering.[95] Almost everyone who had ever given a moment's thought to the NHS (and many who had not) rushed to publish their views on what ought to be done. Conservative ex-Ministers, Think Tanks, professional and other pressure groups and academics, all joined in. In retrospect 1988 stands out not so much as the year in which the NHS celebrated its 40th birthday but as the year of intellectual inflation as reform-mongering became the national obsession. The many and varied manifestos for change fell into two categories. First, there were variations on the theme of replacing a tax-financed by an insurance-based health care system of the 1960s and 1970s (see Chap. 3). Second, there were proposals for improving the use of resources within the NHS by means of organisational change.

Both sets of proposals had one feature in common. They both reflected the influence of American ideas. In the case of those who sought to replace the NHS by an insurance-based system, the influence was clear: the American model of market-based competition.[96] In the case of those who sought organisational change within the framework of the NHS, it was again the impact of American ideas that was striking, and in particular those of Alain Enthoven.[97] His advocacy of an 'internal market' within the NHS, of health authorities buying and selling services to and from each other as well as to and from the private sector, in turn spawned a variety of other proposals: in particular, for health maintenance organisations which, again on the American model, would provide services to those who subscribed to them. There appeared to be a terminal irony in the fact that, after 40 years which had brought a regular procession of Americans to Britain to find out the secrets of the NHS's success, the process was being reversed: the anorexic were seeking a cure from experts on obesity.

Long before the Government's Review was published, however, it became clear that there was no constituency for many of the ideas being floated, especially for those which would have meant radical change in the finance or structure of the NHS. Public support for the NHS did not fall, though worry about standards of service rose:[98] predictably so, given the barrage of professional lamentations. The most popular view was that if the NHS needed more money, it should come out of general taxation. The all-party Social Services Committee, having surveyed the various proposals on offer, came out in favour of cautious and experimental incrementalism.[99] Above all, the medical profession – having raised the spectre of radical reform – took fright. The persistent and strident claims that the NHS was on the point of collapse quickly changed tone. In its evidence to the Government Review, the British Medical Association argued that only 'a relatively small percentage increase in funding' was needed and that it would be 'a serious mistake to embark on any major restructuring of the funding and delivery of health care in order to resolve the present difficulties'.[100] No doubt the BMA was beginning to realise that, as indeed it turned out, the greater the apparent crisis, the stronger the Government's temptation (and ability) to tighten its control over the service providers. Hence, perhaps, the BMA's eloquent testimonial to the NHS, 40 years after having fought its introduction:

While many of the alternative systems have shown superficially attractive features, we have always been led to the inescapable conclusion that the principles on which the NHS is based represent the most efficient way of providing a truly comprehensive health service, while at the same time ensuring the best value for money in terms of the quality of health care. They also enable the cost of health care to be controlled to a much greater extent than has been achieved with other systems, as has been shown by the experience of other countries.

So, faced with the possibility that its campaign of denigration might actually undermine the foundations of the NHS, the medical profession suddenly discovered virtue in precisely the characteristic of the service which had stirred up their ire in the first place: that it was successful in controlling the costs of health care.

Not surprisingly, this was a view finally endorsed by the Government. Very much in contrast to the Royal Commission on the NHS a decade before, the Review was a private affair. It was designed to produce policy options for the Prime Minister, not a public consensus about the NHS. It was, in effect, a three-ring circus revolving around the Prime Minister with ministerial, managerial and medical working groups competing to generate ideas for her. But it soon became apparent that the final product would have to be as much an exercise in political ingenuity as in institutional engineering. Given the expectations aroused by the setting up of the Review, the initial excited speculations that it would come up with some radical wheeze for resolving the periodic funding crises of the NHS, it became essential to find ways of avoiding anti-climax as the realisation dawned that there was no such magic formula: that, particularly for a Government dedicated to containing public expenditure, the NHS was the best instrument of cost-control on offer.

Presentationally, the White Paper that emerged from the Review – *Working for Patients*[101] – turned out to be a triumph. Its radicalism was advertised as much by the Labour Party's determination to present it as a revelation of the cloven hoof of Thatcherism as by the Government's own publicity campaign designed to present it as a millenarian vision of health care in Britain. Never before had any Government document about health care commanded so much space and time in the media. But, leaving aside political hyperbole, *Working for Patients* was remarkable as much for what it did not say as for its actual proposals. A policy reviewed launched in an attempt to devise a new funding system ended up by saying nothing about how to finance the NHS. The Government publicly accepted that there was no way that it could retreat from responsibility for taking political decisions about the level of funding. The Review ended as a re-affirmation of the 1948 settlement and a celebration of the success of the NHS: 'The principles which have guided it for the last 40 years will continue to guide it into the twenty-first century. The NHS is, and will continue to be, open to all, regardless of income, and financed mainly out of general taxation'.

Equally significantly, what had started as a review of funding emerged as a review of organisation. The various proposals fall into two categories. The first set marked the consolidation of the moves towards tighter managerial control that had been so evident in the previous five years and that have already been analysed in this chapter. They represent the final apotheosis, as it were, of managerial rationality – of using central power as a means of achieving greater efficiency and greater control over the providers. The second set marked an attempt, less coherent and more innovative, to move towards competition between providers within the framework of the NHS. They thus represent a break from the past insofar as they also mark the assertion, if only implicitly and tentatively, of a new principle: that public finance of health care need not necessarily be equated with public production – that State responsibility can be divorced from State provision.

So, in the first place, the White Paper announced a spring clean of the managerial hierarchy from top-to-bottom. In a phrase lifted straight from the 1972 Grey Book on the Management of the NHS,[102] providing a reminder of the continuity of ideas over time, the organising concept was that 'delegation downwards must be

matched by accountability upwards'. At the top there was to
be 'a clear distinction ... between the policy responsibilities
of Ministers and the operational responsibilities of the Chief
Executive and top management'. In yet another effort to reconcile
the needs of political accountability with those of managerial
autonomy, the Supervisory and Management Boards became
transmogrified into a Policy Board and a Management Executive
respectively. Below them, the long-standing tensions between
accountability to central government and responsiveness to local
community and professional interests was simply resolved. The
White Paper announced a purge, at all levels and in all health
authorities, of local authority and professional representatives. In
a sense this represents as much a reversion to the principles of the
1974 reorganisation – with their emphasis on the managerial, as
distinct from representative, role – as the logic of what had been
happening in the 1980s. The significant difference, emphasising
the transformation in the political landscape in the intervening
15 years, was that whereas in 1974 the then Secretary of State,
Sir Keith (subsequently Lord) Joseph, retreated under pressure
from the corporate interest groups – and ended up with a
neo-syndicalist solution – by 1989 the government felt no such
inhibitions. On the contrary, the White Paper's strategy in this
respect fitted in snugly with its distrust of both occupational and
local government lobbies: stalwarts of the economic feudalism that,
as noted earlier, the Government was dedicated to destroying.

Not surprisingly, therefore, the other leg of the White Paper's
managerial strategy was to tighten management's grip over health
service providers. So the White Paper proposed that 'every
consultant should participate in a form of medical audit agreed
between management and the professions locally', that all consultants should have job descriptions to cover 'their responsibilities
for the quality of their work, their use of resources, the extent of
the service they provide for NHS patients and the time they devote
to the NHS' and that disciplinary procedures should be streamlined. The secret garden of professional autonomy appeared to be
shrinking to the size of a window box. Moreover, the White Paper
also proposed reform of the distinction awards system which, for
40 years, had served to reflect and reinforce professional values.
It resurrected the notion, first floated by Barbara Castle when
Secretary of State ten years before, that eligibility for awards should
depend on consultants demonstrating 'not only their clinical skills
but also a commitment to the management and development of

the service'. In short, a Conservative Government showed itself prepared to tackle an issue from which a Labour Administration had shied away. It asserted, in effect, that decisions about what counts for good performance by doctors in the NHS could not be delegated exclusively to the medical profession and that determining the currency of accountability in a public service should not be left to the private judgments of the professional providers. In return, the White Paper offered the consultants greater involvement in the processes of management itself. The bargain offered was more influence in managerial decision making in return for less autonomy in medical decision making. Whether or not the profession accepts this bargain, it certainly marks a change in their role and status.

If tightening the managerial grip over the NHS and its providers represented the first theme of the White Paper, attacking institutional rigidities represented the second: the logic being that only a strong managerial framework can allow for flexibility without risking chaos. So, for example, the White Paper announced that individual health authorities could negotiate wage and salary levels in the light of local demands and labour markets: a complete break with the 40 year old tradition of national agreements. Potentially even more important, and certainly more radical, the White Paper moved towards divorcing the finance and the production of health care. It proposed that health authorities would be given budgets determined exclusively by the characteristics of their population, rather than by the number and nature of their institutions, and that they could then decide whether to provide services themselves or to contract for them with other providers, public or private. Indeed the White Paper took one step further towards introducing an internal market. It launched the idea of 'NHS Hospital Trusts': i.e. that NHS hospitals should be allowed to opt for self-government status which would allow them to decide on their own budgets, their own staffing and their own policies, provided always that they could bring in sufficient money from contracts (whether from the public or the private sectors). Ironically it would seem that a Government intent on establishing more managerial control may, at the same time, also be moving towards the creation of provider co-operatives, since one result of setting up NHS Hospital Trusts may well be to strengthen the role of consultants in running them.

The White Paper's plans for general practice reveal similar tensions between different policy aims. On the one hand, there is a re-affirmation of the policies set out in the 1987 White Paper on primary care, discussed above, designed to make GPs more responsive to their patients and more accountable to Family Practitioner Committees. Specifically, the 1989 White Paper took one step further by proposing tighter controls on GP prescribing, including power for FPCs to 'impose financial penalties' on those who refuse to curb excessive prescribing. On the other hand, the Review also launched the idea of GPs as budget holders: that practices with more than 11,000 patients should be given a budget – weighted for the characteristics of their practice population – out of which they would then buy a range of services. These would include out-patient treatment, diagnostic tests and elective surgery but not life-threatening acute care or long-term chronic care. In short, while general practitioners as a whole are to be placed under much tighter managerial tutelage, individual practices would have much more freedom within the constraints of their budgets.

In all this, there is an unresolved dilemma. Can tighter managerial control be reconciled with greater consumer responsiveness? Can promoting the idea of more consumer choice be reconciled with maintaining budgetary discipline? In this respect, the White Paper turned out to be stronger on consumer rhetoric than in explaining just how responsiveness and choice would be promoted by its proposals. If district health authorities contract for services with a particular hospital, it will presumably be on price and quality – so conceivably even limiting consumer choice, since patients might well prefer to go to a different, possibly more convenient, hospital. If general practices are encouraged to move towards large list sizes, in order to become budget holders, the result may be more geographical monopolies, so limiting the ability of consumers to switch their doctors. Conversely, if general practitioners retain the right to refer their patients even to those hospitals where there are no contractual arrangements, leaving it to the districts to pick up the bill, an open-ended financial commitment would be created, making nonsense of budgetary control.

The more contentious and complicated proposals of the White Paper – in particular those for allowing hospitals to opt out and for general practitioners to become budget holders – are not due to be put into practice until 1991. At the time of writing, it is therefore difficult to be sure how enthusiastically and successfully they will be implemented. Much depends on negotiations with the medical profession and developing the information technology required for managerial control. There are also significant silences in the White Paper, in particular about Government's reactions to the recommendations of the 1988 Griffiths Report[103] for transferring responsibility for long-term support for the elderly to local authorities. The overall significance of the Review is therefore best assessed not so much in terms of speculation about its impact on patterns of service organisation and delivery – since it may take the best part of a decade for this to become apparent – but by analysing the general direction and style that it has set for health care.

First, the direction continues to be towards pluralism rather than privatisation. In this respect, little has happened to change the predictions made (Chap. 6, page 193) when the first edition of this book was written. Apart from tax concessions to the over-60s, designed to provide incentives to take out private health insurance coverage, Government policy has not changed. The trend in private insurance coverage therefore looks likely to depend, in the future as in the past, more on social and economic factors than on public policy. Although the proposed quasi-independent hospitals will have an incentive to drum up extra private customers in order to balance their books, the tighter controls over consultants may make it more difficult for them to ply their trade at the expense of NHS commitments.

Second, however, the direction of policy points to the importance of finding a new vocabulary of analysis. The concept of 'pluralism' does not, of itself, capture the full complexity of what is happening. It suggests merely that there will be a greater variety of agencies producing or financing health care. What it fails to convey is that many of the familiar distinctions used to categorise such agencies may no longer be appropriate. So, for example, the boundaries between public and private may be in the process of being shifted or blurred. How, for example, are we to categorise self-governing hospitals occupying a kind of no-man's land between the public and private sectors? Furthermore, the notion of 'pluralism' distracts attention from the fact that by changing the number of agencies involved in health care, we may also be altering their role and function. Most conspicuously, the more the public sector withdraws from the production of services, the greater becomes its responsibility for regulating what is produced by others. This has already happened, as we have seen, in the case of institutional care for the elderly. And the regulatory role of the public authorities is likely to expand greatly if the Government continues to travel along the road mapped out in the White Paper. How else, for example, can the Secretary of State for health ensure that GP budget holders do not discriminate against potentially expensive patients or that self-governing hospitals do not cut corners (and standards) in order to balance their books? In short, the new 'pluralism', or whatever we may choose to call it, will give additional impetus to the transformation of the Welfare State into the Regulatory State.[104]

Third, the new emphasis on flexibility in the organisation of health care draws attention to uncertainty in health policy and the consequent importance of devising organisational structures that can readily adapt: of seeing organised health care as a learning system. Not only is there the genuine unknown: who in the 1970s predicted AIDS, and who can now foretell all likely technological developments? But there are also the difficult-to-calculate implications of the known. For instance, we know that the NHS would have to increase greatly the proportion of school leavers which it recruits – given a dwindling cohort in the relevant age group – to maintain its present nursing strength.[105] But the implications of what happens if it fails to achieve this (as seems highly probable) are far from clear, though they may have a far larger impact on health care delivery than any changes in structure or even financing.

Fourth, it is clear that health policy continues to be a matter of trade-offs between conflicting objectives. The objectives, and the relative weight given to them, may change over time; the conflict, however, remains. So, for example, there has been an emergent consensus throughout the 1980s – reflected as much in the rhetoric of the Opposition Parties[106] as of the Conservatives – on the importance of consumers: an accurate reflection, as argued earlier, of changes in the NHS's environment. But the problem of reconciling consumer demands and choice with budgetary control has not been solved, as we have seen. This is a conflict that has been postponed rather than solved. The strategy of invoking consumer power to balance provider power may help Governments to win battles, but only at the expense of setting up what may be embarrassing expectations for the future.

Lastly, to revert to the theme of the book as a whole, the policy changes of the 1980s underline the importance of developments outside the health care policy arena itself. Some of these are demographic; others are technological; many are social and economic. But, linking and overarching all these, are the changes in the public philosophy: in the way we perceive and define policy issues and our sense of what is possible and feasible. What happens in the NHS inevitably reflects what is happening in other areas. The 1989 White Paper on the NHS was preceded by a Green Paper setting out radical proposals for the reorganisation of the legal profession; the proposal for self-governing hospitals echoes the Government's policy for letting State schools opt out; the proposed internal market for the NHS looks remarkably like the contracting system being devised for universities. To try to predict the future of health care is therefore to take on the much larger task of trying to prophesy what is going to happen to British society as a whole over the next decades. If events since the first edition of this book have taught the author anything, it is that this task is best ducked.

REFERENCES

1. SECRETARY OF STATE FOR HEALTH, *Working for Patients*, London: HMSO 1989, Command 555.
2. JONATHAN GERSHUNY, *Social Innovation and the Division of Labour*, Oxford University Press: Oxford 1983.
3. RUDOLF KLEIN, 'Challenges facing the NHS', *Update*, July 1988, pp. 50–53.
4. A. H. HALSEY (ed.), *British Social Trends since 1900*, 2nd edition, Macmillan: Basingstoke, 1988, Tables 4.1(b) and 10.19.
5. IVOR CREWE, 'Voting patterns since 1959', *Contemporary Record*, Vol. 2, No. 4, Winter 1988, pp. 2–6. The literature on voting patterns, and their significance, is growing rapidly in size and discord. For an overview, see Elinor Scarborough, 'The British Electorate Twenty Years On', *British Journal of Political Science*, Vol. 17, Part 2, April 1987, pp. 219–246.
6. PETER TAYLOR-GOOBY, 'Citizenship and Welfare', in R. Jowell, S. Witherspoon and L. Brook (eds.), *British Social Attitudes: the 1987 Report*, Social and Community Planning Research: London, 1987.
7. CHANCELLOR OF THE EXCHEQUER, *The Government's Expenditure Plans 1988–91*, HMSO: London, 1988, Cm. 288.
8. JOHN CURTICE, 'North and South: the Growing Divide', *Contemporary Record*, Vol. 2, No. 4, Winter 1988, pp. 7–8.
9. OFFICE OF POPULATION CENSUSES AND SURVEYS, 1982, *General Household Survey*, 1982. HMSO: London, 1984. For example, private medical insurance cover in the

Northern Region was *half* the rate that would be predicted on the basis of its socio-economic composition.

10. PETER TAYLOR-GOOBY, 'Privatism, Power and the Welfare State', *Sociology*, Vol. 20, No. 2, May 1986, pp. 228–246.

11. The literature on 'Thatcherism' is vast: for a general review, see DENNIS KAVANAGH, *Thatcherism and British Politics*, Oxford University Press: Oxford, 1987.

12. Originality, it has been said, is a function of forgetfulness: in this case I have, alas, forgotten the source of this phrase.

13. PRIME MINISTER and CHANCELLOR OF THE EXCHEQUER, *Financial Management in Government Departments*, HMSO: London 1983, Cmnd. 9058. This discussed the implementation of policies first set out in: Prime Minister and Minister for the Civil Service, *Efficiency and Effectiveness in the Civil Service*, HMSO: London 1982, Cmnd. 8616.

14. LORD FULTON (chairman), Committee on the Civil Service, *Report*, HMSO: London 1968.

15. Quoted in JOHN URRY, 'Disorganised Capitalism', *Marxism Today*, October 1988, pp. 30–33. The whole issue of the journal is of great interest in its argument that what needs explaining is not Thatcherism as such but the social changes that made it possible. See, in particular, CHARLIE LEADBETER, 'Power to the Person', pp. 14–19.

16. The trend had, of course, been evident for quite some time: see DONALD A. SCHON, *Beyond the Stable State*, Pelican Books: Harmondsworth 1973.

17. D. M. FOX, 'AIDS and the American Health Policy', *The Milbank Quarterly*, Vol. 64, Supplement 1, 1986 pp. 7–33.

18. GEOFF MULGEN, 'The Power of the Weak', *Marxism Today*, December 1988, pp. 24–31.

19. CELIA DAVIES, 'Things to come: the NHS in the next decade', *Sociology of Health & Illness*, Vol. 9, No. 3, September 1987, pp. 302–317; RUDOLF KLEIN, 'Towards a new pluralism', *Health Policy*, Vol. 8, 1987, pp. 5–12.

20. For the distinction between concentrated and diffuse interests, see THEODORE R. MARMOR, *Political Analysis and American Medical Care*, Cambridge University Press: Cambridge 1983.

21. DAVID BUTLER and D. KAVANAGH, *The British General Election of 1987*, Macmillan: London 1988.

22. *The Next Moves Forward* and *Our First Eight Years*, Conservative Central Office: London, May 1987; *Britain will*

win, the Labour Party: London 1987; *Britain United,* Social Democratic Party: London 1987.

23. For example, see SOCIAL SERVICES COMMITTEE Third Report, Session 1980–81, *Public Expenditure on the Social Services,* HMSO: London, 1981, H.C. 324; COMMITTEE OF PUBLIC ACCOUNTS Seventeenth Report, Session 1980–81, *Financial Control and Accountability in the National Health Service,* HMSO: London 1981, H.C. 255.

24. DAVID E. ALLEN, 'Annual reviews or no annual reviews: the balance of power between the DHSS and health authorities', *British Medical Journal,* Vol. 285, 28 August 1982, pp. 665–667.

25. *Information for DHA Chairmen,* Department of Health and Social Security: London n.d.

26. RUDOLF KLEIN, 'Performance evaluation and the NHS', *Public Administration,* Vol. 60, No. 4, Winter 1982, pp. 385–409.

27. CHRISTOPHER POLLITT, 'Measuring performance: a new system for the National Health Service', *Policy and Politics,* Vol. 13, No. 1, 1985, pp. 1–15.

28. PATRICIA DAY and RUDOLF KLEIN, 'Central accountability and local decision-making: towards a new NHS', *British Medical Journal,* Vol. 290, 1 June 1985, pp. 1676–1678.

29. CHANCELLOR OF THE EXCHEQUER, (1988), *op. cit.*

30. ROY GRIFFITHS (chairman), *Report of the NHS Management Inquiry,* DHSS: London 1983.

31. CHRIS HAM, 'The NHS – travelling without map or compass' *Health Service Journal,* 14 April 1988, pp. 412–413.

32. See the evidence given by Tony Newton, Minister of State for Health, to the SOCIAL SERVICES COMMITTEE Session 1987–88, *Resourcing the National Health Service: Minutes of Evidence 8 June 1988,* HMSO: London, H.C. 264-XII.

33. SIR ALEC MERRISON (chairman), *Report of the Royal Commission on the National Health Service,* Para. 19.31, HMSO: London 1979, Cmnd. 7615.

34. PATRICIA DAY and RUDOLF KLEIN, 'The mobilisation of consent versus the management of conflict: decoding the Griffiths report' *British Medical Journal,* Vol. 287, 10 December 1983, pp. 1813–1816.

35. See evidence given by Griffiths to the SOCIAL SERVICES COMMITTEE, First Report, Session 1983–84, *Griffiths NHS Management Inquiry Report,* 1984, HMSO: London, H.C. 209, Q. 431.

36. All the quotations come from a valuable study of NHS managers: Philip Strong and Jane Robinson, *New model management: Griffiths and the NHS*, Nursing Policy Studies Centre, University of Warwick: Coventry, July 1988.

37. A sign of the times was the publication of TONY BUNBURY and ANGUS McGREGOR, *Disciplining and Dismissing Doctors in the National Health Service*, Mercia Publications: Keele 1988; see also 'Summary dismissal of consultants', *British Medical Journal*, Vol. 298, 7 January 1989, pp. 10–11.

38. JOHN YATES, *Why are we waiting?*, Oxford University Press: Oxford 1987.

39. NATIONAL AUDIT OFFICE, *Use of Operating Theatres in the National Health Service*, HMSO: London, 1987, H.C. 143. See also CHRIS HAM (ed.), *Health Care Variations*, King's Fund Institute: London 1988.

40. PATRICIA DAY and RUDOLF KLEIN, *Accountabilities*, Tavistock Publications: London 1987.

41. For a general overview, see OFFICE OF HEALTH ECONOMICS, *Measurement of Health*, OHE: London 1985 and CLAIRE GUDEX, *Qalys and their use by the Health Service*, Discussion paper No. 2. Centre for Health Economics: University of York, 1986. For a specific study, see MARTIN BUXTON ET. AL., *Costs and Benefits of Heart Transplant Programmes*, HMSO: London 1985.

42. See, as an example of early interest in clinical budgets, IDEN WICKINGS, *The Effects of Presenting Management Information to Clinically Accountable Teams*, Health Information Unit, Brent Health District: London, May 1975.

43. CHRIS HAM, ROBERT DINGWALL, PAUL FENN and DON HARRIS, *Medical Negligence*, King's Fund Institute: London 1988.

44. PATRICIA DAY and RUDOLF KLEIN, *Inspecting for Quality*, Bath Social Policy, Paper No. 12, Centre for the Analysis of Social Policy: Bath 1988.

45. WALTER HOLLAND and ELLIE BREEZE, 'The Performance of Health Services', in M. KEYNES, D. A. COLEMAN and N. H. DIMSDALE (eds.), *The Political Economy of Health and Welfare*, Macmillan: Basingstoke 1988; PAUL KIND, *Hospital Deaths – the missing link*, Discussion Paper No. 44, Centre for Health Economics: York, 1988; for a discussion of negative performance indicators, PATRICIA DAY and RUDOLF

KLEIN, 'Quality of institutional care and the elderly', *British Medical Journal*, Vol. 294, 7 February 1987, pp. 384–387.

46. N. BUCK, H. B. DEVLIN and J. N. LUNN, *The Report of a Confidential Enquiry into Perioperative Deaths*, The Nuffield Provincial Hospitals Trust/The King's Fund: London 1987.

47. NOEL TIMMINS, 'Hospitals to audit work or to risk losing doctor posts' *The Independent*, 29 December 1988.

48. For a general review of the development of acute private health care, see JOAN HIGGINS, *The Business of Medicine*, Macmillan: Basingstoke, 1988.

49. INDEPENDENT HOSPITALS ASSOCIATION, *Survey of Acute Hospitals in the Independent Sector, 1988*, IHA: London, July 1988.

50. WILLIAM LAING, *Laing's Review of Private Healthcare, 1988/89*, Vol. 1, *Acute Healthcare*, Laing & Buisson: London 1988. This invaluable annual survey has been drawn on throughout for basic information about the private sector.

51. J. P. NICHOLL, N. R. BEEBY and N. T. WILLIAMS, 'The Role of the Private Sector in Elective Surgery in England and Wales, 1986', *British Medical Journal*, Vol. 298, 28 January 1989, pp. 243–247; J. P. NICHOLL, N. R. BEEBY and B. T. WILLIAMS, 'Comparison of the activity of short-stay independent hospitals in England and Wales, 1981 and 1986', *British Medical Journal*, Vol. 298, 28 January 1989, pp. 239–243.

52. DAVID HORNE, *Public Policy Making and Private Medical Care in the UK since 1948*, PhD thesis, University of Bath, 1986. This brings together evidence on both consumer attitudes and the lack of correlation between 'inadequate' NHS funding and demand.

53. OFFICE OF POPULATION CENSUS AND SURVEYS (1984) *op. cit.*, p. 160.

54. WILLIAM LAING, BRIAN BRICKNELL, ROY FORMAN and NANCY SALDANA, *Keeping the lid on costs?*, IEA Health Unit Paper No. 4, IEA Health Unit: London 1988.

55. Calculated using figures drawn from William Laing (1988) *op. cit.*

56. PATRICIA DAY and RUDOLF KLEIN, 'Towards a new health care system?', *British Medical Journal*, Vol. 291, 2 November 1985, pp. 1291–1293.

57. LAING (1988), *op. cit.*, Vol. II, *Long Term Health and Social Care*.

58. For the market in nursing homes, see DUNCAN LARDER, PATRICIA DAY and RUDOLF KLEIN, *Pricing the Nursing Home Industry*, Bath Social Policy Paper No. 9, Centre for the Analysis of Social Policy: Bath 1986; for the structure of the private acute hospital sector, see Independent Hospitals Association (1988), *op. cit.* The latter has been characterised in the 1980s by the declining share of charitable organisations (from 59 per cent of all beds in 1979 to 45 per cent in 1988) and independent hospitals (from 20 per cent to 13.5 per cent) and the rising share of for-profit groups (from 8 per cent to 40 per cent), among them some of the leading American corporations in this field.

59. PATRICIA DAY AND RUDOLF KLEIN, 'Residential care for the elderly: a billion pound experiment in policy-making', *Public Money*, March 1987, pp. 19–24.

60. AUDIT COMMISSION, *Making a Reality of Community Care*, HMSO: London, 1986.

61. In particular, SIR ROY GRIFFITHS, *Community Care: An Agenda for Action*, HMSO: London, 1988.

62. G. C. FIEGEHAN, 'Income after Retirement', *Social Trends No. 16*, HMSO: London, 1986, pp. 13–18. For a critical view of this interpretation, see PAUL JOHNSON AND JANE FALKINGHAM, *Intergenerational Transfers and Public Expenditure on the Elderly in Modern Britain*, Centre for Economic Policy Research Discussion Paper No. 254, London, 1988.

63. DUNCAN LARDER, PATRICIA DAY and RUDOLF KLEIN, *Institutional Care for the Elderly: the geographical distribution of the public/private mix in England*, Bath Social Policy Paper No. 10 Centre for the Analysis of Social Policy: Bath, 1986.

64. PATRICIA DAY and RUDOLF KLEIN, 'Maintaining standards in the independent sector of health care', *British Medical Journal*, Vol. 290, 30 March 1985, pp. 1020–1022.

65. For an analysis of a succession of inquiries into conditions in NHS hospitals, see J. P. MARTIN, *Hospitals in Trouble*, Basil Blackwell: Oxford 1984; for more recent evidence, see DAY and KLEIN, *Inspecting for Quality, op. cit.*

66. For this analysis, I have relied on the excellent account in KATE ASCHER, *The Politics of Privatisation*, Macmillan: Basingstoke 1987.

67. NATIONAL AUDIT OFFICE, *Competitive Tendering for Support Services in the National Health Service*, HMSO: London, April 1987, H.C. 318.

68. ROBIN G. MILNE, 'Competitive tendering in the NHS', *Public Administration*, Vol 65, No. 2, Summer 1987, pp. 145–160.

69. S. BIRCH, 'Increasing Patient Charges in the National Health Services: a method of privatizing primary care', *Journal of Social Policy*, Vol. 15, Part 2, April 1986, pp. 1634–185.

70. SOCIAL SERVICES COMMITTEE Fifth Report, Session 1987–88, *The Future of the National Health Service*, HMSO: London 1988, H.C. 613.

71. PATRICIA DAY and RUDOLF KLEIN, 'Controlling the gate-keepers: the accountability of general practitioners', *Journal of the Royal College of General Practitioners*, Vol. 36, March 1986, pp. 129–130.

72. For the most recent analysis of general practice see DAVID WILKIN, LESLEY HALLOW, RALPH LEAVEY and DAVID METCALFE, *Anatomy of Urban General Practice*, Tavistock: London 1987.

73. SECRETARY OF STATE FOR SOCIAL SERVICES, *Primary Health Care: an agenda for discussion*, HMSO: London 1986, Cmnd. 9771, Chapter 2, para. 2.

74. JOHN WHEATLY, *Prescribing and the NHS: the Politics of the Limited List*, M.Sc. thesis, University of Hull, 1985. In what follows I have drawn on this excellent study for both analysis and quotations.

75. SECRETARY OF STATE FOR SOCIAL SCIENCES (1986), *Primary Health Care: An Agenda for discussion, op. cit.*

76. SOCIAL SERVICES COMMITTEE First Report, 1986–1987 Session, *Primary Health Care*, HMSO: London 1987, H.C. 37.

77. SECRETARY OF STATE FOR SOCIAL SERVICES, *Promoting Better Health*, HMSO: London 1987, CM 249.

78. PATRICIA DAY and RUDOLF KLEIN, 'Weighing up opposing models of health care', *Health Service Journal*, 8 May 1986, pp. 618–619.

79. PATRICIA DAY, *Women Doctors*, King's Fund: London 1982.

80. JANE LEWIS, *What Price Community Medicine?*, Wheatsheaf Books: Brighton 1986; SARAH HARVEY and KEN JUDGE, *Community Physicians and Community Medicine*, King's Fund Institute: London 1988.

81. DANIEL M. FOX, PATRICIA DAY and RUDOLF KLEIN, 'The Power of Professionalism: Policies for AIDS in Britain, Sweden and the United States', *Daedalus*, 1989 forthcoming.

82. CHARLES WEBSTER, *The Health Services Since the War Vol. 1: Problems of Health Care: The National Health Service Before 1957*, HMSO, London, 1988.
83. SOCIAL SERVICES COMMITTEE First Report, Session 1987–88, *Resourcing the National Health Service: Short Term Issues*, HMSO, London, 1988, H.C. 264, Table A.
84. SOCIAL SERVICES COMMITTEE Fourth Report, Session 1985–86, *Public Expenditure on the Social Services*, HMSO, London, 1986, H.C. 387. The Minister concerned, Mr. Barney Hayhoe, did not survive long.
85. DEPARTMENT OF HEALTH AND SOCIAL SECURITY, *Health care and its costs*, HMSO, London, 1983.
86. SOCIAL SERVICES COMMITTEE First Report, Session 1987–88, Vol. 11, *Minutes of Evidence*, pp. 96–108.
87. PATRICIA DAY and RUDOLF KLEIN, 'Future Options for Health Care', in SOCIAL SERVICES COMMITTEE, Session 1987–88, *Resourcing the National Health Service: Memoranda laid before the Committee*, HMSO: London 1988, H.C. 284-IV, pp. 48–51.
88. For a good account of events and issues, see NICHOLAS TIMMINS, *Cash, Crisis and Cure*, The Independent: London, 1988.
89. CENTRAL COMMITTEE FOR HOSPITAL MEDICAL SERVICES, *NHS Funding: The crisis in the acute hospital sector*, BMA: London, 1988.
90. DHSS evidence to the SOCIAL SERVICES COMMITTEE, Third Report Session 1987–88, *Minutes of Evidence, op. cit.* p. 105.
91. NATIONAL ASSOCIATION OF HEALTH AUTHORITIES, *NHS Economic review, 1987*, NAHA: Birmingham, 1987.
92. For an American perspective on this, see HENRY J. AARON and WILLIAM B. SCHWARTZ, *The Painful Prescription*, The Brookings Institution: Washington, 1984.
93. For example, SIR BRYAN THWAITES, *The NHS: The End of the Rainbow?*, Institute of Health Policy Studies: University of Southampton, 1987.
94. 'Clarke opens new financial chapter', *British Medical Journal*, Vol. 297, 12 November 1988, p. 1217.
95. For a review of the various proposals and a bibliography, see JOHN BRAZIER, JOHN HUTTON and RICHARD JEAVONS (eds.), *Reforming the UK Health Care System*, Discussion Paper 47, Centre for Health Economics: York, September 1988.

The politics of the National Health Service

96. For example, carrying the torch first lit in the 1960s by the
     Institute of Economic Affairs, DAVID GREEN, *Everyone a
     Private Patient*, London: IEA Health Unit 1988.
97. ALAIN C. ENTHOVEN, *Reflections on the management of
     the National Health Service*, London: Nuffield Provincial
     Hospitals Trust 1985.
98. 'The public speaks out on the NHS', *Health Service Journal*,
     19 May 1988, pp. 556–557.
99. SOCIAL SERVICES COMMITTEE Fifth Report Session 1987–88,
     The Future of the National Health Service, London: HMSO
     1988, H.C. 613. The appendices to these reports give a
     comprehensive picture of the variety of proposals on offer.
100. 'Evidence to the government internal review of the National
     Health Service', *British Medical Journal*, Vol. 296, 14 May
     1988, pp. 1411–1413.
101. SECRETARY OF STATE FOR HEALTH (1989), *op. cit.*
102. DEPARTMENT OF HEALTH AND SOCIAL SECURITY, *Manage-
     ment Arrangements for the Reorganised National Health
     Service*, London: HMSO 1972, Para. 1.5(e).
103. SIR ROY GRIFFITHS (1988), *op. cit.*
104. PATRICIA DAY and RUDOLF KLEIN, 'The business of
     welfare', *New Society*, 19 June 1987, pp. 11–13.
105. MARGARET CONROY and MARY STIDSTON, *2001 – The
     Black Hole*, NHS Regional Manpower Planners' Group,
     May 1988, Mimeo.
106. See for example ROBIN COOK, *Questions of Health*, London:
     Labour Party 1988.

INDEX

Dawson report, 4, 6
Department of Health and Social
    Security, 66, 78, 79, 93, 97, 98,
    110, 116, 122, 124, 126, 127,
    128–9, 130, 131, 133, 135
(DHSS)
    centralisation, 200–4
    managerial changes, 208–14
    and private sector, 214–22
    strategies, national, 206
Directory of Organisations for Patients,
    and Disabled People, 116
District General Hospitals, 73, 74, 75,
    99, 136
District Health Authorities, 135, 136,
    138, 139, 187
District Management Teams, 93, 95, 98
doctors, 21, 22, 49, 114–15
    see also family doctors, general
    practitioners, junior hospital
    doctors, medical profession
Down's Children's Association, 116

Ely inquiry, 80, 96, 130
Enthoven, A., 236
Executive Committees, 22, 57
Executive Councils, 97, 138, 162
Expenditure Committee, 126, 127,
    171–2

Family Doctor Charter, 87, 88, 89
family doctors, 87
Family Practitioner Committees, 97, 98,
    131, 133, 138, 162, 163, 226–7,
    241
Financial Management Initiative, 198
Foot, Michael, 1
Fowler, N., 204, 224
Fox, Sir Theodore, 114
Fraser; Sir Bruce, 66
Fulton Committee on the Civil Service,
    65
funding, 201–4, 228–35

Gaitskell, Hugh, 34
General Medical Council, 161–2
general practitioners, 3, 13, 14, 15, 16,
    23–4, 44, 53, 54–6, 87–9,
    88–9, 154, 162

General Practitioners' Association, 87
Germany, 167
Godber, Sir George, 44, 54, 66, 164
Goodman, Lord, 123
Griffiths, Sir R., 208, 209
Guillebaud Committee, 34, 35, 39, 40,
    43, 52, 53, 57, 58, 73, 133, 134

Hawton, Sir John, 10, 42
Health Advisory Service, 213
health authorities, 93–6, 110, 137,
    187–8
health care
    changes in policy for, 105–6, 117,
        124
    conflict of ideas concerning, 7
    consensus of ideas concerning, 2–7
    depoliticisation of, 63–4, 76
    efficacy of, 167–8
    efficiency in, 64–5
    expansion of, 65–6
    financing of, 190
    local government and, 5, 6
    new developments in, 63–4, 68
    politics of, 9, 12, 33, 62–3, 153
    policy aims and values of, 184–5
    prevention and, 171–4
    social factors and, 174–7, 191–2
Health Centres, 14, 15, 16, 22, 23,
    88–9, 97
health education, 172
health insurance, 4–5, 6, 7, 71, 134
health service administrators, 55
Health Service Commissioner, 84, 163
health service workers, 21, 22, 43, 69,
    111, 130, 188–9
Health Services Board, 123, 134
Heath, Edward, 65
Hill, Charles, 24
Hospital Activity Analysis, 84
Hospital Advisory Service, 80
hospital building, 62–3, 76, 78, 81,
    110, 126
Hospital Consultants' and Specialists'
    Association, 89, 121
Hospital Management Committee,
    21–2, 47, 48, 49, 57, 77, 78, 96, 97
Hospital Plan for England and Wales,
    73, 74, 75, 77, 78, 80, 81